Ruttl V. Kirk

TRAUMATIC INCIDENT REDUCTION (TIR)

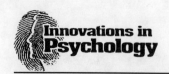

INNOVATIONS
in PSYCHOLOGY

Series Editor
Charles R. Figley, Ph.D.
Florida State University

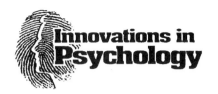

Innovations in Psychology

TRAUMATIC INCIDENT REDUCTION (*TIR*)

Gerald D. French
Chrys J. Harris

CRC Press

Boca Raton   London   New York   Washington, D.C.

Library of Congress Cataloging-in-Publication Data

French, Gerald D.
    Traumatic incident reduction (TIR) / by Gerald French and Chrys Harris.
        p. cm. — (Innovations in psychology series)
    Includes bibliographical references and index.
    ISBN 1-57444-215-5 (hbk.)
    1. Post-traumatic stress disorder—Treatment—Handbook, manuals, etc. 2. Psychic
trauma—Treatment—Handbooks, manuals, etc. I. Harris, Chrys. II. Title. III. Series.
    RC552.P67F74 1998
    616.85′21—dc21
                                    98-3810
                                      CIP

© 1999 by CRC Press LLC
St. Lucie Press is an imprint of CRC Press LLC

No claim to original U.S. Government works
International Standard Book Number 1-57444-215-5
Library of Congress Card Number   98-3810
Printed in the United States of America   2 3 4 5 6 7 8 9 0
Printed on acid-free paper

DEDICATION

We dedicate this volume to the memory of Lt. Col. Chris Christensen (Ret). Chris was a kind, gifted, and truly remarkable man. He died suddenly and unexpectedly, at far too young an age, on the morning of October 29, 1992, in the course of pursuing his formal duties, then in Europe, arranging for the transshipment of humanitarian aid desperately needed by the people of Eastern Europe following the breakup of the Soviet Union. We have quoted Chris below, and some of the ingenuous words with which he described his selfless work with TIR introduce each of the chapters of this book.

Chris was a student in the first-ever TIR Workshop, taught by French in 1989 at the Institute for Research in Metapsychology in Menlo Park, CA. A veteran who had spent two years in combat in Vietnam, frequently involved in what were called "unconventional" solo operations, Chris had gone to work for the Idaho Department of Employment in Lewiston subsequent to his retirement from the army, coming eventually to work exclusively with jobless vets as a Disabled Veterans Outreach Program Specialist.

In the course of that work, he discovered posttraumatic stress disorder and that his clients were not the only ones who had it, though his own symptoms did not prevent him from working full-time. Chris heard about TIR and came to be trained in it in a roundabout fashion.

A co-worker in Lewiston who had himself heard about it on a radio interview with another vet (conducted by Florida psychologist Robert Moore) described what he had heard to Chris, but could remember only the fact that the program had originated in Florida. With remarkable perseverance, Chris managed to track down first the correct radio station and then Dr. Moore himself. Moore in turn was able to refer him to the vet he had interviewed by telephone in California. To make a long story short, Chris came to California, learned TIR, and from then until the day he died, he employed it unselfishly, as a labor of love, with virtually every needing, hurting person he encountered. Given the nature of his chosen work, those folks were legion.

Of the period before he left for Europe, he later wrote, "When I arrived at Job Service in Lewiston, Idaho, back in April 1985, there were in excess of 150 disabled veterans on the rolls, seeking employment. I worked with those people up until the time that I went to California to receive my TIR training, and so we had close to five years that I worked very hard with those folks to put 'em to work and keep 'em in jobs. I would say at the time that I went to California, I still had 120 of those people on the roles, seeking employment. With the skills learned through TIR training—and I'm talking about the one-week, 40-hour intensive course that Gerald gave me and Lori Beth—I would estimate that I have worked with close to 60 of those people, anywhere from two hours to 20 hours at the most, the average probably running around 14 or 15 hours. And out of those 60 people that I worked with on TIR, I had two—that's one, two!—left on the roles, seeking employment, when I left Idaho for Germany three weeks ago."

We have quoted Chris at the beginning of Chapters 1 through 10 with some of the ingenuous words he used to described his work as a "Wildcat" TIR facilitator. Chris sent French a tape he'd made one evening shortly after his arrival in Germany. He dictated it while sitting on a single bed in a small hotel room, and the quotes preceding each of the chapters were taken from a transcript of that tape, previously published in a newsletter of the Institute for Research in Metapsychology and quoted herein with permission.

Christensen's unbridled enthusiasm for and delight in communicating about the power of the tool he had discovered were a constant source of inspiration to French, Gerbode, and others working with TIR and related techniques who, in their efforts to "spread the word" about these promising approaches, sometimes felt a bit like voices crying in the wilderness. On being notified of Chris' death, Gerald wrote the poem that follows. It was read as the eulogy at the memorial service held for him in Germany:

The Wildcat

I lost the best of friends today, and weeping, write.
I hope he knows; I'm sure he does.
His passing was not natural
To those of us who loved him and whose lives he touched;
We truly rage against the dying of that bright and hope-filled light.
Chris, you were the "Wildcat" to me.
I can't recall for sure just how you came to bear that name—
That of a bear is much more nearly what your hug was like.
I do remember that you said you killed a wildcat once—with reverence—
And "Wildcat" was what you called the work you came to do
So selflessly and well,
Toward the ending of your days.
You did not come to us for company.
You never feared to be alone ...
Or, if you did,
Your courage never failed you.
In your youth, ofttimes alone,
You faced and fought a mortal enemy ...
And killed ...
And you were injured in the killing.
And then, in finding healing for yourself,
Discovered in yourself the gift of healing others.
The sword that you had wielded so well
Became a ploughshare in your gentle, battle-hardened hands.
Before you left us for another life,
You carried peace to scores of sufferers
Who came to you with hope, because they'd heard
That you had something
That could help them past the rough spots.
You did ...
And in your name, I'll see it used by someone else
To help me past the rough spot
Of your passing.
Farewell, my friend.
Go in peace, and so return.

ACKNOWLEDGMENTS

There are a number of individuals who deserve acknowledgment for their invaluable aid to us in writing and putting this book together.

French: I must begin by acknowledging Frank A. ("Sarge") Gerbode, friend, philosopher, renegade psychiatrist, and the man most responsible for having put together the subject of metapsychology, out of which TIR and a host of other valuable approaches to healing and growth have arisen.

A relative handful of caring and accomplished friends, therapists, and facilitators made Gerbode's work possible through their generous contributions of time, insight, and experience. Steven Bisbey's work was essential, but a list of others whose efforts and support were critical to the development of this subject at many points along the way includes, as well, Lori Bisbey, Helen Burgess, Nancy Day, Teresa Descilo, Brian Grimes, Hildegard Jahn, Karyn Kuever, Aerial Long, Ragnhild Malnati, Robert Moore, and Marian Volkman. Gerbode has cited others in his own work. I thank Larry Voytilla for his excellent figures, some of which he modified at short notice for this book.

I am grateful to my teachers at Palo Alto's Institute of Transpersonal Psychology, whose gentle and salutary influence can be perceived particularly in the chapter on communication.

With enormous respect, I wish to express my gratitude to Charles Figley, without whose interest, support, and encouragement, this book would never have seen the light of day. His faith inspired me, as it has a host of others.

Finally, if one is fortunate, fate graces his life with true friends and wise companions. Those who know Chrys Harris and my wife, Bia Oliveira, will confirm that I have been fortunate indeed.

Harris: At the outset I need to acknowledge Gerald French, Charles Figley, and CRC Press for extending to me an invitation to co-author this volume, which becomes a part of the "Innovations in Psychology Series". I shall forever be grateful for the opportunity.

I want to thank my father for his reassurance and support as I began this process. He passed away on September 8, 1997, and was a pillar in my life—sometimes he held me up, sometimes he came crashing down on my head. I recall an episode of the original *Star Trek* series where the underlings on a distant planet considered their overlords as *the givers of pain and pleasure;* this was my father. Although he bore witness to the beginning, he will not bear witness to the end of this endeavor; he will always have some responsibility for my part of it.

A number of individuals contributed e-mail responses in an effort to make our book come together. Charles Figley, Joyce Carbonell, and Lori Beth Bisbey account for the bulk of the research that exists on TIR. Each put forth effort to communicate with us about their research—past and pending.

One of my marriage and family therapy students at Converse College, Jeff Barnett, deserves mention. His interest in emotional trauma and neurolinguistic programming has resulted in many interesting conversations that encouraged me to keep my theories and beliefs in perspective and to remember they are not dogma.

Lastly I recognize my wife, Judy. Her dedication and sacrifice were instrumental in providing me with time and resources to take on and complete this project.

EDITORIAL NOTE BY THE SERIES EDITOR

Telling one's story, reenacting significant conflicts, and composing a dialogue with oneself leads to understanding about past events. This working through of troubling, distressful memories is the hallmark of effective psychotherapy. Creative literature is full of stories about emotional journeys of remembering, recovering new information, formulating new conclusions about the past, and, in doing so, acquiring a sense of peace and fulfillment. Psychologists have known for some time that bearing witness to the life experiences of a client is helpful.

Carl Rogers in the early 1940s was one of the first psychologists to challenge the theories of psychoanalysis and other interpretive and categorizing treatments. Rogers' nondirective therapy, through unconditional positive regard for the client, became a major contribution to helping clients reach peace of mind. Rogerian counselors act more like companions and facilitators in the client's journey toward self-understanding and greater life satisfaction. Rogers believed that all creatures strive to make the very best of their existence, and that if they fail to do so, it is not for lack of desire.

Rogerian therapists employ reflection. Reflection is the mirroring of emotional communication: if the client says, "I feel like dirt!", the Rogerian may reflect this back to the client by saying something like, "Seems as if you feel that life's getting you down." In doing so, the therapist means to communicate to the client that he/she is listening and cares enough to wish to understand. Reflection must come from the heart; it must be genuine and congruent.

Too often, however, in an effort to reflect what the client is saying, the Rogerian therapist or facilitator has tended to direct the client to the therapist's worldview. It is difficult not to do so. But there may be other ways for the therapist to show the client that he/she is listening and cares.

In conversations with both clients and friends, we interact. We give and take. Even when we attempt to remain neutral, we are not. In most instances, this is what is expected. Yet there is a very special population—people who suffer as a result of past experiences—which benefits most from being given the space to speak without evaluative interaction.

This is one of the major precepts of Traumatic Incident Reduction (TIR). At no time during a session do the protocols of TIR permit the therapist/ facilitator to interfere in any way with the client's viewing of and report on the trauma being addressed—as by offering any sort of comment, leading question, interpretation, observation, suggestion, or reflection. The intensity of the helper's interest is conveyed by listening alone, and by the simple acknowledgment that follows only upon the client's having said everything he/she had to say. The elegant simplicity of the TIR procedure itself is counterbalanced to a significant degree by the tightly focused interest and restraint that this approach demands of the therapist who would use it.

TIR is the latest in the CRC Press Innovations in Psychology Book Series. The Series Editorial Board and I are quite pleased to offer this book to the field of psychology and to other professions that work with clients haunted by traumatic memories. We established the series to stimulate innovation in the psychological sciences. Of special interest are the acute problems of traumatized clients. In the first book in the series, *Burnout in Families: The Systemic Costs of Caring,* family psychologists shared their findings and clinical innovations to help families struggling with secondary traumatic stress.

The second book of the series, *Energy Psychology: Explorations at the Interface of Energy, Cognition, Behavior, and Health,* offered a new branch of psychology. It linked the current theories with the new paradigm of energy systems and their effects on emotions and behaviors. This included, but was not limited to the psychological effects of highly stressful events.

TIR offers a new way of approaching an old problem: how to resolve the emotionally charged memories that surface in dreams, flashbacks, and behaviors or life patterns that the client finds debilitating. The old way involved analysis, reflection, or some other clinical technique that required the therapist to sort through what the client was saying and to attempt to help the client reach insight. As you will see in the coming pages, TIR adopts the new paradigm of psychotherapy: it is brief, client-centered, and client-paced. Its clinical successes are clearly defined: traumatic memories are cognitively reprocessed, and the client is desensitized.

We urge readers to write to the Editorial Board of the Innovations in Psychology Book Series. You can reach us through the publisher, CRC Press. We look forward to learning about your experiences in using TIR, suggestions for improving subsequent editions of this book, and ideas about books for the series.

Charles R. Figley, Ph.D.
Series Editor
Professor and Director
Florida State University Traumatology Institute
Tallahassee, Florida, USA

FOREWORD

In beginning these notes, I wish to acknowledge the authors for having taken the highly unusual step of asking me—an absorber rather than a dispenser of therapy, a client rather than a colleague—to write this foreword. Their request is very much in keeping with the philosophical orientation of TIR, an approach to dealing with posttraumatic and other painful conditions that is truly, even radically, client-centered, as you will discover.

Originally, having read a number of my e-mail posts* to a forum focused on trauma, Gerald asked me if I'd be willing to describe some of my own experiences with TIR as a contribution to this book. Initially, he and Chrys had told me they considered including my reflections as a brief case history, written from the viewpoint of a client. Following some discussion on the telephone, however, Gerald asked me if I'd be willing to tackle the ocean instead of the swimming pool, and actually to set forth what follows.

I had a brief moment of panic. The panic was very real, and probably based on a long history of self-doubt, feelings of unworthiness, passivity, and an obsessive perfectionism. That its intensity dwindled to nothing in the space of no more than perhaps ten seconds is the first of a great number of positive changes that have recently occurred in my life that I believe stem directly from my experience with the procedure that this book describes.

I first came across traumatic incident reduction (TIR) on the internet in early 1997. I had been researching various concepts of traumatic bereavement, had read some insightful papers by two of the leading researchers on childhood trauma (Bruce Perry and Bessel van der Kolk) and was deeply involved in correspondence with Dr. Holly Prigerson at the Yale School of

---

*These were posts on the subject of my own recovery, by way of TIR, from the trauma that characterized my childhood.

Biomedicine and Dr. Katherine Shear of Western Psychiatric Institute and Clinic concerning their theories and research into what was then being termed *Traumatic Grief*. Truth be told, what I was really engaging in was an attempt to find a path toward my own healing; toward ending the pain, confusion, and uncertainty that had kept my true sense of myself, my abilities, my fulfillment, and any real pleasure in life at bay for the previous 40 years. When I was six years old, my mother died of a cerebral hemorrhage, suddenly and unexpectedly. Her death left me with unresolved mourning, morbid and overwhelming grief, and a profound sense of subconscious guilt, exacerbated by the fact that her death was never discussed, explained, or dealt with at the time that it happened. There was no funeral, no grave site or memorial, and very few mementos of her existence. Because of that, and because of the fact that my relationship with her before her death was also ambivalent (and co-dependent, due to her own untreated depression) it is perhaps not surprising that some of my pathology included an inability to accept the reality of her death at a core level. Thus, I developed an unconscious tendency to search for the lost object of attachment, coupled with learned helplessness, compulsive care-giving, low self-esteem, self-destructive behavior, abandonment anxiety disorders, and an inability to express anger, accompanied by profound irrational fear. My father, too, was suffering depression and a host of other devils of his own. In consequence, however unintentionally, he was given to shaming and other forms of psychological abuse, thus creating yet another layer of trauma.

My family's history includes bipolar disorders (with concomitant hospital confinements and suicide attempts) and a disproportionate share of depressive disorders, on both paternal and maternal sides, some of which are probably partially genetic in origin. My own more recent history consisted of six major depressive episodes of long duration, requiring medication, and five losses of significant relationships, each of which I perceived as utter abandonment. In sum, then, as you might imagine, I had a great susceptibility to triggering of very painful negative affect throughout my life by any circumstance bearing even the faintest resemblance to earlier and seemingly similar traumata. I had been in ongoing psychotherapy for the past 25 years with three very competent therapists—Freudian, Jungian, and Cognitive/Behavioral—and I had been on antianxiety and antidepression medication, including Valium, Flurazepam, various tricyclics and, most recently, SSRIs.

Needless to say, after slipping into another deep depression following yet another loss of a significant relationship in the fall of 1997, with all the familiar accompaniment of the associated massive triggering of emotional affect from earlier traumas, I was ready to consider the possibility of a different approach to my worsening condition. Several days before my 47th birthday, I embarked on a course of TIR— one that led me, in a matter of a very few days, to a place of complete resolution and to a kind of peace I had never experienced. The experience enabled me to effect changes in my self and my perception of the world that I and those who know me well have had no hesitation in labeling dramatic.

I employ the term "dramatic" in full awareness of the fact that its use may engender a certain skepticism among therapists jaded by anecdote. So be it. I could find no better word in *Webster's Dictionary*, Second Edition, unabridged, which defines it as: "of, or pertaining to, the drama; vivid; expressed with action," and of drama: "a composition, usually in prose, arranged for enactment and intended to portray the life of a character, or to tell a story, with dialogue tending toward some result." The process of TIR contains all of these elements. It allows one to tell one's "story", to reenact it, to compose a dialogue with oneself that seemed inevitably, to me, to lead to a very significant result: the action of the "drama" resolving into a much-desired outcome. In my case, the outcome has been healing, peace, satisfaction, fulfillment, and the cessation of often unbearable pain and distress.

TIR gave me the ability to resolve and eliminate all the major negative affects surrounding my mother's death and the subsequent additional traumas. It gave me the ability finally to acknowledge and accept the reality of that death and loss, and I am now in the process, with other members of my family, of creating the actual, physical, previously unfinished grave-marker destined to become her memorial. It gave me profound relief from all the unconscious feelings of guilt on both an inexplicable emotional level and a very real and present cognitive level.

TIR has allowed me to restructure a very deep and impairing belief system that had kept me from the joys and fulfillment that I now know I deserve and desire and have begun to attain. It has restored to me my self-esteem and heightened my confidence, else you would not be reading this. Recently, I have experienced several situations any one of which, at any time in the past, would have triggered intense feelings of abandonment, rejection, anxiety, or apprehension in me. Since my few sessions of TIR and Unblocking (that's another remarkable tool you'll learn about in this book), I have met those situations positively and optimistically, and without any of the negative emotional charge that would have dominated my responses in the past.

With what was for me astonishing rapidity, TIR ameliorated all aspects of my depressive symptoms, both mental and physical. It has allowed me, for the first time in 25 years, to feel wholly comfortable in discontinuing all antidepressant medication (despite my concern over the fact that earlier this year my father tried to do the same and ended up in his worst depression ever, followed by an almost-successful suicide attempt, four months of hospitalization, extensive ECT, and now a tenuous recovery). Following TIR, with medical approval and encouragement, I have stopped taking a daily 50 mg of the SSRI, Paxil.

TIR has allowed me to accept and undertake increased responsibility in my life and in my community and to embark on a new career of which I had previously only dreamed. The support that I have received from my community has been equally rewarding. TIR, in fact, has given me back my life.

Do I think these changes will be long-lasting and permanent? Yes.

Do I know why? Yes.

Could I explain why? Yes...but the authors of this book do it better than I could.

Do I think that I will ever be clinically depressed again? Probably not.

Do I think I'm the exception rather than the rule in the degree of transformation I have experienced? Possibly, but then I've lately encountered a lot of impressive anecdote out there suggesting that my experience with TIR is not that uncommon.

Recently, in the Traumatic-Stress Forum begun on the internet by Charles Figley, there was extended discussion of a series of questions regarding if and how trauma might actually be "cured" (a word I've seen enclosed by quotation marks much more often than not when used by professionals in the context of traumatic sequelae). One of the participants in the Trauma List posted the following:

> My guess is that clients are brimming with their own wisdom regarding what is in the way of their cure, and that likewise, many are just waiting for therapists to ask some simple questions. Which brings me to another question: what keeps therapists from asking these questions?

I am convinced that the therapist/facilitator using TIR is asking, perforce, some of the most important of these very simple questions, and (if (s)he has been well trained) asking them in such a way that a client like myself can glean enormous insight, wisdom, and relief in the flow of his/her own answers.

In reviewing the many thoughts that others have recently shared with me concerning the question of whether all trauma can be cured, I have concluded that the answer is, "Yes". I do believe all nonphysical trauma can be cured, and that the cure can be as complete and permanent as we desire it to be. I also now know that the cure need be neither as difficult nor as time-consuming as most of us (clients and therapists alike) have in the past been led to believe.

This book describes the basic techniques, structures, and communication skills necessary for the effective administration of TIR. The authors also describe Unblocking, another valuable procedure that can enable you as a therapist or facilitator to address situations where your client's memory of a specific traumatic event seems to be unavailable, or where repetitive traumas seem to have occluded the ability of the client to know what areas of life most need to be addressed.

Since I hope I am speaking from the viewpoint of your client, or as one trying to put myself in his/her shoes, I urge you to be open to the possibility that a remarkably high percentage of clients know what they need in order to change, and will find it by themselves if allowed to look in the absence of certain kinds of proffered "help" and "support".* I believe that any one of us (who meets certain prerequisites) is capable of tracing unwanted feelings, sensations and perceptions back to their origins and, in the simple act of "viewing" those origins, of eliminating their pain and of changing forever for the better, their bitter cognitive associations.

Again, it is possible to learn to ask a remarkably few questions that open up the possibility of healing; simple questions like, "tell me what happened". The authors of this book stress the therapeutic value of a therapist's *not* asking, or saying, much else; of granting the client the empowerment that comes (I can attest) from having confronted his or her own devils and nightmares—uninterpreted, unevaluated, and unaided—and from having had the freedom to reach his or her own conclusions concerning their true nature and significance.

A therapist I spoke with recently addressed the issue well:

> In any case, with trauma, we are apparently not dealing with any total or permanent structural changes, since many people seem to completely get over the negative "charge" associated with the events. So, "cure" seems to me to be a reasonable word to describe there no longer being an

---

* "Help" and "support" which, in my extensive experience as a client, I have all too often found to be an integral part of the therapist's armamentarium.

ongoing problem. If the charge is gone, why not use the word "cure"? If we remember that the same incident may be experienced as traumatic by one person and not another, then we conclude that the trauma is in the experience, not the event. Similarly, it is not in the memory. So, if memories are still there without the traumatic charge (and the traumatic charge doesn't come back) then I'd call that "cured". I think part of the problem has been our limited expectations based on our previously limited tools. People have grown to expect only to feel "less bad", or to feel bad less often. I think that if we set our sights on anything less than cure, we will wind up settling for less than we need to.[*]

I want to acknowledge the authors of this book for placing, as all facilitators do, such a large amount of trust in their clients—their "viewers"—and for allowing me (without ever even having met me) the very healing opportunity to write this foreword. If this description of my own experiences and of the transformations I have undergone as a result of my own personal and profound encounter with TIR has served in any way to whet your appetite for more, I shall have performed a valuable service.

We may not have a solution for many of the illnesses in this world. We may not have a cure for cancer or AIDS or arthritis. However, I believe that we have, with TIR, a cure for trauma-induced mental and emotional complications, even severe ones. With this in mind, I urge you to use the knowledge and the wisdom contained in this book to the best of your abilities. I think it will make quite a difference in the world—a place that I now truly enjoy and look forward to being in for quite some time.

Peter Shefler
Emerson Point, Maryland, USA

---

[*] Quoted by permission from a post on the Traumatic-Stress Forum by Harry D. Corsover, Ph.D.

PREFACE

We have written this manual for therapists, counselors, psychiatrists, clinical social workers, and other helpers. In part, our intent has been to provide a more detailed and accessible reference manual than has heretofore been available for use by those working with Traumatic Incident Reduction (TIR). Our hope is also, however, that the work will serve as a practical and convincing introduction to TIR for those unfamiliar with the approach.

The first description of TIR was contained in Frank Gerbode's book, *Beyond Psychology: An Introduction to Metapsychology,* published in 1988.* Although we have drawn extensively on that excellent work, our focus here has largely been a practical one. We encourage readers who wish to acquire a detailed understanding of the background and theoretical and philosophical underpinnings of TIR and related metapsychology-based procedures to consult that earlier volume.

By definition, TIR as a therapeutic tool lends itself perhaps most obviously and readily to addressing and resolving the mental and emotional sequelae of known traumata: rape, combat, childhood sexual abuse, natural disasters, traumatic bereavement, and the like. For that reason, we have dwelt for the most part on its use with survivors of such events. That fact notwithstanding, we urge readers to bear in mind the wealth of anecdotal evidence suggesting TIR's effectiveness (in its "Thematic" form—see Chapter 2) in resolving as well a litany of symptoms and conditions representing a substantial percentage of the subject matter of *DSM-IV.* This includes such diagnostic categories

---

* *Beyond Psychology* can be obtained through the Traumatic Incident Reduction Association (TIRA), 13 NW Barry Road, Suite 214, Kansas City, MO 64155-2728; phone: (816) 468-4945; fax: (816) 468-6656; e-mail: tira@tir.org; <http://www.tir.org>.

as adjustment disorders, acute stress disorder, bereavement, dysthymic dis-order (chronic depression), major depressive disorder, anxiety disorder, som-atization disorder, sexual abuse, a variety of phobias, and more.

We have withheld nothing we are aware of in the way of essential data concerning the TIR procedure and its competent administration, and an intelligent and caring reader might well encounter a significant—even remarkable—level of success in the use of TIR working only from this book. No book, however, can ever substitute for training with an experienced instructor. Responsible use of any nontrivial technique demands it, and should you decide to incorporate the approach into your repertoire, we urge that you seek out and attend a professional workshop.*

---

* The authors of this book offer such workshops, as do a number of other instructors certified by TIRA. Dates and venues of TIRA-certified workshops held in the U.S. and overseas are regularly posted at <http://www.tir.org> and at <http://www.healing-arts.org/tir>.

CONTENTS

ABOUT THE AUTHORS

Gerald D. French

I was born in San Francisco in 1941, three weeks before the bombing of Pearl Harbor. Shortly after the U.S. entered the war, my mother, a gifted painter, went to work as a volunteer nurse's aide at Stanford Hospital, then in the City, where my father, an M.D., was head resident and had been placed on the essential teaching staff list. I've believed all my life that I can recall being held in my nurse's arms to look out over the darkened city during a blackout in the early months of the war, despite having been told that I was too young to remember that and that it must be my imagination.

I grew up in the city I was born in, a place of whose beauties I stood in awe, even as a very young child. One of my most treasured recollections of my earliest years is of riding with my father just at sunset in the lovely old DeSoto convertible in which, *mirabile dictu,* he made housecalls. We were driving north on the Great Highway toward Playland-at-the-Beach, an amusement park that stood throughout my childhood like a gaudy sentinel guarding the western approaches of the Pacific to Land's End and the Golden Gate. Some strange arrangement of the summer's fog advancing on the coast reflected the rays of the dying sun off the bottoms of the cloud mass, and the ethereal light pouring over the cold, grey-green breaking ocean was like no light I had ever seen before. It made me feel like crying, or maybe cheering. I recall, distinctly, wondering if other people ever felt that way just from looking at something. My father, too, was struck by it, for he stopped the car by the side of the road, took my hand, and ran with me across the deserted highway to the windswept seawall where we sat and watched the brief remainder of that stunning sunset.

For the most part, I didn't like school, and I came to truly loathe it during one particular two-year stint—my sophomore and junior years at the Middlesex School in Concord, MA. I manifested sufficient unhappiness during my stay there that my parents at one point actually arranged an appointment for me with a therapist in Boston. I remember the session clearly. The therapist's first words were, "You're smoking a cigarette...you're insecure!" I decided on the instant that the man was an idiot, though more to be pitied than censored. Following this auspicious start, he asked me what I dreamed about. I told him about a dream I'd had once in which I was hanging from a tightrope strung across our neighbor's yard in San Francisco while a large black dog, snarling and barking, repeatedly leapt up at me from below and tried to eat me. The therapist had a field day with that dream, as I recall. I continued to despise school, and never did have a second session with the therapist. That was the only conventional "therapy" experience I ever had.

In the fall of 1964, at age 22, I married Rosamond Miller, a Wellesley graduate that I had dated for two years while an undergraduate at Harvard. We lived for a year and a half in Oakland, while I got halfway to a Master's in architecture at UC, Berkeley before deciding that that field was not one in which I would ultimately be happy.

During that time, years when Vietnam was becoming a sinkhole for the youth of a number of countries, including ours, my draft board ordered me to a physical. Some weeks subsequent to that event, I received on the same day not one but two letters from the army. The first one I opened congratulated me on having been found 1A, the second expressed regret at my having been determined to be 4F on account of asthma. Following at least one and perhaps as many as two seconds of deep reflection, I tore up the former, framed the latter, and hung it over our mantelpiece. Such was my Vietnam experience.

Gifford Pinchot IV, a college classmate of mine, came to visit in San Francisco while I was midway through a Master's Fellowship in Early Childhood Education at SF State College (now University) in 1969. Gifford had become fascinated with Dianetics and Scientology—the Church (CofS) founded by LaFayette Ronald Hubbard. Gifford convinced first my wife and then me that they were worthy of a look. I took a look that lasted nearly 15 years. During the first two of those years, I directed and taught in two classrooms of the Headstart Program in East Palo Alto, dubbed by the press at the time as the "murder capital of the U.S.". Over the ensuing years, my wife graduated from Santa Clara Law School and became (eventually) Chief Counsel at NASA, Ames. I became the father of two wonderful and utterly beloved children—a son, Lindol, and a daughter, Seri. As well, I became a highly trained "auditor", administrator, and Deputy Director of the Palo Alto Mission of the CofS under my oldest boyhood friend, Frank Gerbode.

Gerbode was and remains a renegade psychiatrist, a Stanford graduate who studied philosophy at Cambridge, then attended Yale Medical School and returned to the west coast where he completed a psychiatric residency at Stanford before becoming involved with the CofS. Our time together in the Church is probably worth a novel some day. Meanwhile, suffice it to say that the two of us left the group in 1984. The separation was not without a certain drama, though certainly no tears were shed by either the Church or us, its apostates. We took with us the desire to help others and the interest in matters of the spirit that had led us to explore it in the first place.

After our exodus, Gerbode founded and I became Director of a small institution in Menlo Park—the Institute for Research in Metapsychology (IRM)—renamed the Traumatic Incident Reduction Association (TIRA) in February 1997 and under a new director since March of that year. For the past 14 years, we and other active members of the Institute have worked to discover, develop, and promulgate replicable, teachable tools and procedures that we believe to have the potential to reduce significantly the sum of human suffering in the world. My own contribution to this work included speaking and teaching at a great many professional conferences and workshops in North and South America, Europe, Japan, and Australia, as well as maintaining the membership roles and editing and producing the Institute's Newsletter from the mid 1980s until 1997.

Among the tools we developed at the Institute during that period was TIR,[*] the principal subject of this book, and, certainly the best-known product of the Institute to date. As one of the developers of TIR, I instructed the first formal TIR workshop teaching its use in the late 1980s, co-authored the

---

[*] In his book, *Beyond Psychology: An Introduction to Metapsychology* (1988, IRM Press, Menlo Park, CA), Gerbode outlines the philosophical tenets cn which TIR and related metapsychological techniques and approaches are based, and describes at length the origins and background of the subject. Though most were first described in print by Gerbode in his book (above) and in several journals and instruction manuals published by the Institute, the procedures themselves were developed over the years by a number of people with whom Gerbode consulted frequently, including Steven Bisbey, C.T.S., and Lori Beth Bisbey, Ph.D., C.T.S. (England), Helen Burgess (NY), Nancy Day, C.T.S. (MO), Teresa Descilo, M.S.W., C.T.S. (FL), Gail Gerbode (CA), Brian Grimes, C.T.S. (CA), Hildegard Jahn, Dipl. Soz., C.T.S. (Germany), Karyn Kuever, M.S.W., C.T.S. (WA), Aerial Long, M.A. (OR), Ragnhild Malnati, M.S.W., C.T.S. (MD), Robert Moore, Ph.D., C.T.S. (FL), Marian Volkman, C.T.S. (MI), and myself.

manual used today by certified TIR instructors to give the workshop, and continue frequently to instruct four-day workshops in the method.

My wife and I separated in 1989 and subsequently divorced, and I married a second time in 1991, once again to an immensely strong and capable woman, but at the same time, one who could hardly be more different from my first wife, Rosamond, the attorney—she of Wellesley and the great American heartland of southern Ohio. Beatriz Maria de Castro Oliveira was born and raised in Sao Paulo, Brasil. Like mine, her father was an M.D. Bia is an intuitive; a "seer", perhaps, is the best word for her. She works with the tarot, and astrology, and numerology, and has abilities and a connection with the universe that I don't pretend to understand but for which experience has forced me to develop a respect that borders at times on awe. Bia has an enormous clientele in Brazil and, of late, a growing one in northern Italy and on both coasts of the U.S. as well. During the first year I knew her, I regarded her work with a sort of benign tolerance bordering on cynical indifference, a fact which causes me great shame when I think of it today.

One night, after a late dinner, I found myself talking to her sadly about how much I missed my father, who had died of Alzheimer's disease in my arms some years earlier. "He was so kind", I said to her, "and so many people loved him. God, I hope he's OK now."

"He's fine", she said. "He's here."

"He's *here*?" I asked. "*Now*??"

"Yes," she said. "He says to tell you he's fine, and not to worry."

"How ... do you know?" I asked, wanting terribly to believe her, but unable to crack the barriers of my own indifferent cynicism. (Lord, show us a sign....)

"Because he's *speaking* to me", she said patiently.

"What is he saying now?" I asked.

"He's telling me to ask you if you remember the fog, and the sunset, and the ... convertible."

I think she may never have said or even heard the word "convertible" in English before that moment, and hence her hesitation. Certainly she'd never heard me say it. My father and I were the only two people on earth who knew about our having watched that sunset.

Through my tears, I thanked her.

My work with TIR and trauma and its transformation has been informed by such events, and I am now once more a student working toward another Master's, this time in Counseling Psychology at the Institute of Transpersonal Psychology in Palo Alto.

Chrys J. Harris

Until shortly after my 20th birthday, my life was not unlike that of a great many other young American males of my generation. In March 1968, that changed, abruptly and drastically. I was involved in a military helicopter training accident that left me a paraplegic. Although the U.S. Army and, later, the Veterans Administration, got me through the physical issues, there were mental and emotional ones that persisted. I don't believe I would ever have met the criteria for a diagnosis of posttraumatic stress disorder (one that at the time, of course, did not exist) but I did have residual issues that I certainly didn't deal with appropriately. Although I attempted to confront my demons, I found that at some level they remained out of reach and unapproachable.

Years later, I read a wonderful, unpublished paper by Jack Russell in which he discussed the pros and cons of sealing over one's traumatic experience. Although Jack didn't recommend it, I decided to attempt to do just that (Jack, if you read this, I'm sorry!). I stuffed my residual issues into a metaphorical ziplock "baggie" and put it on a suppressed shelf—seemingly out of mind, out of perception.

Truth be told and unbeknownst to me at the time, it was probably those ziplocked issues that brought me into the field of psychotherapy generally and specifically led to my work with PTSD. As the year after my injury progressed, it became apparent to me that I was becoming addicted to soap operas and needed to do something with my life other than watch TV and feel sorry for myself. I turned to school. The GI Bill provided me with an undergraduate education in psychology (B.S., 1973) from Wofford College in Spartanburg, SC and the VA vocational education program granted me a Master's in school psychology (M.A. in Ed., 1975) from Wake Forest University in Winston-Salem, NC.

After laboring unhappily as a school psychologist for five years, I went to work for the VA with Vietnam veterans and their families, identifying and treating combat-related traumas for the most part. It was during this period that my interest in PTSD (newly identified and legitimized through the American Psychiatric Association [1980]) began to blossom. Training in dealing with PTSD was not broadly available at the time due to the newness of the diagnosis. After three-and-a-half years with the VA, it became very clear to me that I needed to seek out whatever knowledge did exist if I were ever to enable my clients to do more than simply cope half-heartedly with the consequences of their traumata. I looked for and found the leading nonmedical authority on PTSD—Charles Figley, then at Purdue University—and went back to school. My doctoral work there (Ph.D., 1988) under Dr. Figley lead me to a post-doctorate at the University of Pennsylvania medical school for my psychotherapy preparation as a marriage and family therapist.

I first encountered TIR at an annual meeting in 1994 of the International Society for Traumatic Stress Studies (ISTSS) during a presentation given by Frank Gerbode and Gerald French and moderated by Charles Figley. Charles had spoken with me earlier, suggesting that I might want to hear the Gerbode and French presentation on TIR as he felt it would offer something new, exciting, and challenging to my views of treating PTSD. Figley's enthusiasm was more than enough of a "hook" to assure my attendance.

During that talk, I began to feel that I was experiencing a turning point in my life as a therapist, and the passage of time since then has confirmed that belief. The presentation given by Gerbode & French—the essence of which is thoroughly addressed in this volume—offered me the first suggestion I had ever encountered that PTSD might not only be treated but fully resolved ... and in a stunningly short space of time. The method they presented was concise, it made good sense, and the taped sessions they showed were unlike any I had ever seen in terms of both degree of positive outcome and of the speed with which it was obtained.

At the time, I and many of my colleagues tended to regard some form of burnout or secondary traumatization (also referred to as compassion stress or compassion fatigue, depending on the severity) as an all-but-inevitable consequence of working with a heavily traumatized clientele. During his part of the presentation, French wondered aloud if it did not make better sense to imagine that such negative consequences were inevitable only when working *ineffectively* with such clients. That thought gave me pause. As the two men took turns speaking and showing videos of TIR sessions, I found the term "cure" coming unbidden to mind. I resisted it, and my background and training prevented me from dwelling on it, but I became so enthralled that I found myself wanting more than the relatively brief presentation could offer.

The icing on the cake was Charles' declaration that he and Joyce Carbonell had initiated a study at Florida State University concerning TIR and several other approaches to the rapid resolution of trauma, collectively dubbed "the power therapies" by numerous enthusiasts.

After the presentation, I sought out Gerald during a poster session he and Gerbode were hosting on TIR. Truthfully, I could not get excited about the poster display; I had too many questions to ask and things I wanted to talk about. Gerald spent more time with me than he should have (ignoring some of those who wanted to discuss the poster issues) which whetted my desire to know even more. I left the conference with newfound hope, and assurances from Gerald that he would send me information on TIR.

During the next year or so, I attended other presentations by Gerbode and French, and in May 1995, Charles brought the major spokespeople of the four "power therapies" together at Florida State University to hold a symposium with invited guests. The idea was to present the archetypes and discuss these innovative models. I was privileged to be invited and in attendance. During this conference, I had uninterrupted time with Gerald to ask still more questions, to learn more, to compare TIR with the other highly touted models for treating PTSD, and as it turned out, to build my excitement to a fever pitch. I made arrangements to go to California to be trained.

I arrived in Menlo Park for the training in February 1995, led by French—who was assisted by Ragnhild Malnati, a certified and very gifted TIR facilitator/therapist from Washington, DC. The intensive four-day workshop more than fulfilled my expectations. I spent the time immersed in TIR with Gerald, Ragnhild, and my fellow trainees, and as luck would have it, had even a little time to spend with Dr. Gerbode, whose wisdom added clarity to what I had learned.

For me, one of the most important results of the training, and certainly the most immediate, occurred on the last of the four days in menlo park. That afternoon, we students were divided into working dyads and given the chance to use the TIR procedure with each other under real session conditions. Recall my "baggie on the shelf"? I had become sufficiently comfortable by that time, with both my partner in the dyad and with Gerald's supervision, so that I took a chance, brought it down from the "shelf", and opened it. By the end of the session, the baggie was empty and I found myself all but overwhelmed with utterly unexpected insight and understanding. In just more than an hour, I had achieved a feeling of relief and liberation that I found astonishing, and that has remained with me ever since.

In the three years subsequent to that remarkable experience, I have worked with TIR in addressing a myriad of issues with clients in my private practice, primarily in the resolution of traumatic events and panic disorders, but also as a successful intervention in dealing with obsessive-compulsive and generalized anxiety disorders. I have also worked with Gerald at a national TIR training session in Charleston, SC where my job was to speak to the question of how to integrate TIR into traditional therapeutic models.

In writing my portion of the text that follows, and in continuing to absorb TIR and its implications—technically, philosophically, and therapeutically—I realize that I have more to learn, and I find the prospect to be an exciting one. I base the faith I have developed in the transformative power of TIR on my own remarkable experience as a "viewer", and on the continuing confirmations of its efficacy provided to me regularly by my clients. The validity of TIR has only recently begun to be substantiated by quantitative research (see the Epilogue), but I am certain that more such research will be forthcoming, and that the results will continue to cast this approach in a most favorable light.

Regardless of the current scarcity of scientific facts and data, I am grateful to Gerbode, the Bisbeys, Gerald, and the many others who have made this elegant implement available to the therapeutic community, and am reminded of Thomas Huxley's observation that, "In scientific work, those who refuse to go beyond fact rarely get as far as fact."

THERAPY FOR THE RESPONSE TO EMOTIONAL TRAUMA

1

It is amazing how hard it is to recall the individual, and his or her traumatic incident and how they unraveled in our sessions. It seems as though the training that I received is extremely successful in allowing my viewers to walk away without their heavy pictures "sticking" on me. As a result, I have found that it is, in some cases, difficult even to remember the names of the people that I have worked with over the last, oh, almost two years now.

Another thing that has become very evident to me in working with TIR is that I have become much more tolerant in my understanding of what a traumatic incident is. I've realized that what is traumatic to one may well not seem traumatic to another, and that what may seem insignificant to me can be a mountain of crap to another. It is amazing to see what might be, by my definition, a very insignificant thing, cause a tremendous amount of pain — real pain — and emotional discharge in another. That's been a very positive learning experience for me, one that says, "Don't mess with the system!" TIR works ... as long as you don't mess with it. Good stuff!

It is amazing how relaxed and tolerant I've become, too, when observing intense emotional discharge take place in a viewer during a session of TIR. While a viewer is in the bottom of the pit, groveling, snot-running, etc., I've come to know full well that this is [just] a process that takes place, the end result of which is going to be just ... beautiful! And when they come back up out of that crap and look at you, clear-eyed, and say, "Wow! Thanks!" ... Well, it's just wonderful stuff.

Another thing I've learned is that it's impossible to assist a person through the TIR processes and mentally jump ahead to a "logical" conclusion. If there is one thing that I have found, it is that if I lose concentration during a session—if my "shield" goes down—and part of my mind jumps forward to a conclusion, I can almost rest assured that that conclusion will be the wrong one when it all washes out. That again says to me: Be very confident in the process of TIR itself. Let the process run its course. I may well tend to allow things to continue longer than I normally would, or than I would normally feel comfortable in doing, but I have found that by allowing TIR to run its course, even if it is longer than where I think it might want to go, I find that the end result tends to be much more satisfying, much more clear in the viewer's mind. And as a result, the success at the end of it is just short of phenomenal.... *

THE INDIVIDUAL RESPONSE TO EMOTIONAL TRAUMA

According to van der Kolk & McFarlane [30, p. 3], "experiencing trauma is an essential part of being human." If this is true, the stress response that commonly follows such an experience should be considered an inevitable part of humanity. Indeed, one of the authors of this book [19] has suggested elsewhere that acute victimization** resulting from exposure to a traumatic event is an expected consequence and is a prominent part of the recovery process. It requires the psychological work that involves assimilation and accommodation of the traumatic experience into idiosyncratic models of self and the world. It is this idiosyncratic model of self and the world that determines how each of us will cope with a traumatic experience.

The term idiosyncratic suggests an individually unique methodology of sorting the world. The perceptual system through which each of us experiences the world, including our mental constructs of it, is idiosyncratic;

---

* This quote is continued at the beginning of each chapter. It is reprinted with permission from the Fall 1992 issue of the *Newsletter of the Institute for Research in Metapsychology* (IRM, now TIRA), Vol. V, Issue 3.

** Frequently, if not typically in the trauma field, the terms victim and survivor are used interchangeably. Figley (1985) suggests, however, that it is useful to distinguish between them—the victim being dysfunctional due to the traumatic experience, while the survivor is functional in spite of it. There are a number of individuals and groups who make a clear distinction between the two and prefer to be called survivors rather than victims due to the stigma attached to the perception of the latter as dysfunctional. In this book we make the distinction in order to clarify and maintain a focus on the concept of psychological movement from victim to survivor.

colored by our experiences, the system in turn renders each of us unique [20]. The human sensory-based perceptual system is composed of vision, hearing, smell, taste, and touch. In addition, there is a sixth sense that Lewis & Pucelik [24] recognize: our emotional feelings or our kinesthetic sense. These six senses are the only way to discern our world [20].

The present authors find useful the idiosyncratic model of self and the world based in part on the insightful work of Janoff-Bulman [22, p. 5] who proposes that we have, within us, a conceptual system that "developed over time, provides us with expectations about the world and ourselves." She asserts that we have a foundation of assumptions that provides the rudimentary basis for our beliefs about ourselves, our world, and the relationship between the two. Further, she contends these assumptions are relatively inaccessible and resistant to our own introspection. The implication of this assumptive world is that it is a distinctive loupe through which we perceive all that we are and all that the world is to us. In spite of this enlightenment, we still do not understand why we perceive as we do.

Korzybski [23, p. 750] observed that "a map is not the territory." In fact, a map is a representation of the territory and humans have representational systems, like maps, in which we depict ourselves and our world. In order for these representational systems to function, they have to be both biased and resistant to change. Janoff-Bulman [22, p. 27] describes a "cognitive conservatism" where perception is considered to be an inferential process that gathers data, filters them through a biased lens, and interprets them in an personal and unique manner. She calls the lens a schema, and it is the mechanism through which new data are filtered and assimilated into preexisting theories. The result is how the present authors believe our perceptions are derived—we filter incoming data through our idiosyncratically biased loupe or schema, and then form opinions, beliefs, values, and attitudes, as well as create and change theoretical perspectives.

Resistance is an important part of the schema as it acts as an authority, allowing accommodation of the data that are harmonious with the schema and rejecting all or part of the data which are not compliant This may account for what appears to be a selective loss of information when victims are asked to recall the traumatic events or experiences.

As a result of the idiosyncratic perception, Janoff-Bulman [22, p. 89] suggests a traumatic experience will test "our fundamental assumptions... [and] ...challenge these core schemas." For some, following an exposure to a traumatic event, there are insufficient data in the core schema to call upon or data that are inconsistent or dissonant with the lessons the trauma would teach. When this is the case, the assumptive world comes "tumbling down" [22, p. 89]. In other words, the core assumptions cannot assimilate and accommodate the traumatic experience so attempts to do so cease; and posttraumatic stress disorder ensues.

POSTTRAUMATIC STRESS DISORDER

Trauma research dating back to the late 1970s (for excellent reviews of a historical perspective on psychological trauma see Trimble [29] or van der Kolk et al. [31]) suggests that although 50 to 90% of victims move into survivorship, many never suitably recover from their traumatic experiences. Ten to fifty percent of all trauma victims remain traumatized, moving only from acute to chronic victimization. This is where recovery has ceased; this is posttraumatic stress disorder (PTSD).

Probably the most comprehensive definition, as well as symptoms, of PTSD can be found in the *Diagnostic and Statistical Manual of Mental Disorders, Fourth Edition (DSM-IV)* [1]. The *DSM-IV* actually describes two forms of posttraumatic stress. The first is called acute stress disorder (ASD). We can use its definitions and symptoms to verify that an individual is experiencing acute victimization. This is the expected, albeit predictable, phase of recovering from the trauma that we mentioned earlier in this chapter. The second description is that of the chronic stress response called posttraumatic stress disorder, or PTSD. This diagnosis requires that the following criteria are met:

1. Actual or threatened death, serious injury, or threat to the physical integrity of self or others
2. The victim's intense fear, helplessness, or horror
3. Persistent reexperiencing of the traumatic event
4. Persistent avoidance of any stimulus associated with the traumatic event
5. Persistent symptoms of arousal

For a minority of individuals there are major barriers to overcome when doing the work involved in psychological trauma resolution. Most individuals have the skills and resources to surmount these barriers but a select few do not. The key question is: Why do some pass through and beyond a traumatic experience while others do not? In other words, Why are some schemas able

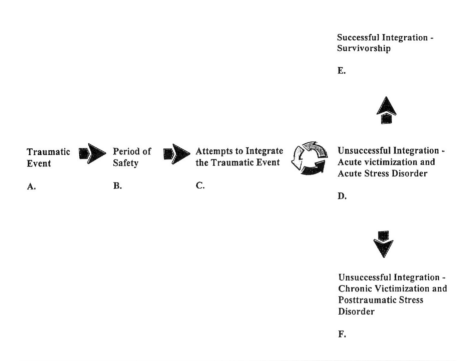

Figure 1   Etiology of posttraumatic stress disorder. (Adapted with permission from Ref. 18, p. 103.)

to assimilate and accommodate a traumatic experience while others are not? We do not have this answer yet. But we do have an idea of how the trend of psychological trauma recovery—both successful and unsuccessful—develops (see Figure 1).

When the traumatic event (phase A) occurs, the victim's behaviors and emotions are related to the actual event and are occurring concurrently with or within the event. These are the behaviors associated with making it through the event and its consequences. We all saw victims of the Oklahoma City bombing of the Murrah Federal Building on television as they moved about, some in a daze, some with purpose, some yelling, and some quiet. Each was doing what (s)he needed to do to make it through the aftermath of the experience. An enormous array of behaviors are expected under such circumstances, ranging from appropriate (even predictable) to clearly inappropriate and unpredictable.

Then, following the traumatic event, there is a period of safety (phase B). This concept was introduced by Horowitz [21] to suggest there is a time when the victim can say it is all over. During this phase, the actual traumatic event is over but the psychological consequences remain and must be integrated within the idiosyncratic self and the world. It is here that many victims cease to make progress in their quest to integrate the traumatic experience. If a victim is unable to reach or sustain a sense of safety—to experience a traumatic event as past, and fully completed—then the process of recovery becomes stagnant. Rape victims suggest that the event is not over because "The trial is yet to come," "The perpetrator is in jail but could get out," or "The perpetrator has not been caught." A combat veteran reports, "This can never be over." An automobile accident victim adopts the belief that not only is (s)he vulnerable, but that "doom is just around the corner." A mill worker who lost a hand in a machine states, "I just have a sense that my family and I are no longer safe."

In these cases, the victims do not continue the process of moving from victim to survivor. In other words, they cannot or do not move to the next phase; they stop trying to assimilate and accommodate the traumatic experience and move into the chronic phase of PTSD (phase F). However, if they can reach a belief that they are safe and the trauma is over, they will move on. At this point, it is important to note that the psychological work involved in the rest of the phases (from phase C on) involves the exertion of memory—the representation of the traumatic event and not the actual event itself. In fact, we might say PTSD is a memory management problem.

During phase C, the actual work of assimilating and accommodating the memories of the psychological trauma into the individual schema takes place. At this point, the victim is at a place where a DSM-IV diagnosis of ASD can be made (assuming it is within a 30-day time period). In phase D the effort to integrate becomes unsuccessful—an evolution that all victims go through. The present authors have never encountered a case without an unsuccessful integration. (In other words, a case in which integration of a traumatic event was both successful and immediate.) As a matter of fact, the loop between phases C and D is the crux of the process of integration. Here, the trauma experience attempts to integrate with the existing schema and the operation of assimilating what is consistent with the schema, rejecting what is inconsistent, and accommodating the results takes place—all to create new schema.

If the integration is successful, the victim moves to survivorship in phase E. Figley [11] suggests this survivorship is relatively easy to recognize. The trauma victim marks the move from victim to survivor by answering five survivor questions with little or no negative affect. The survivor can say:

1. What happened
2. Why it happened
3. Why (s)he acted as (s)he did at the time of the traumatic event
4. Why (s)he has acted as (s)he has since the traumatic event
5. What will happen if the traumatic event happens again

The present authors suggest these questions bring the survivor to an understanding of the present schema under which (s)he is operating. In essence, the victim makes sense of the traumatic experience and, by allowing it to fit with the self and the model of the world, becomes stable and completes the integration process by assimilating and accommodating the event into the schema.

On the other hand, if energy flags over time, and as a result of the increasing time and decreasing energy, the victim's conscious and unconscious attempts at integration fail, then those efforts cease. Here the victim has integrated all (s)he could into the schema without resolving all the consequences of the trauma. As a result, the loop between phases C and D ceases. The acute victim moves into and tacitly accepts the identity of chronic victim, and PTSD (phase F) ensues.

TRAUMATIC INCIDENT REDUCTION AND TRAUMA RESPONSE

The therapeutic goal for a victim with PTSD is to move from the chronic stage of victimization back into the previously unsuccessful acute stage since that is where assimilation and accommodation occur. Referring again to Figure 1, the victim is moved from phase F back to the phase C/phase D loop.

Gerbode [14]* states that what must be assimilated and accommodated from a traumatic incident are one's reactions to the incident—including one's thoughts, sensations, feelings, and perceptions. He further states that for any trauma to remain emotionally charged and unresolved, "part or all of a traumatic incident [must remain] uninspected" (p. 436). This means the victim has incompletely perceived the traumatic incident and has not made sense of it.

To inspect, perceive, and understand the traumatic experience stored in memory, Gerbode [14] describes a method of sequentially going through the

---

* See Gerbode's work in this reference for a philosophical orientation to TIR.

experience a number of times (cf., moving back to the C/D loop in Figure 1). He calls this archetype traumatic incident reduction (TIR). TIR is based on the premise that there is a primary traumatic root incident in one's experience that other subsequent traumatic incidents, or sequents, are dependent upon. We can better understand the root and sequent structure from the perspective of Pavlov's classical conditioning.

Pavlov originally experimented by presenting dogs with meat while ringing a bell to elicit a salivation response. In the original set of conditioning trials, Pavlov presented dogs with meat to elicit salivation. This is the root incident because it includes an action, consequences of the action, and a distinct beginning, middle, and end to the event. At this point, the meat or the bell elicits salivation. What if Pavlov had then gone through a new set of conditioning trials to pair another sound with the bell? At the end of such trials, the new sound would presumably elicit the salivation. This new set of conditioning trials (actions, consequences of actions, and a beginning, middle, and end) would combine to become a sequent. The sequent would elicit the same salivation as the root, even though it is removed in time and the stimulus is different from the initial bell. Reasonably, Pavlov could have gone through several sets of conditioning trials so that several stimuli would elicit the salivation response. Each of these sets of conditioning trials would be an additional sequent. They are inextricably linked to the initial set of conditioning trials. In other words, the sequents are inextricably linked to the root.

Trauma symptoms, therefore, are "powered by" the emotional charge associated with a root incident, one which may be far removed in time from the most recent experience of the symptom. Moore [25] points out that as Pavlov paired the bell with the meat, the pairing of one stimulus with another ad infinitum creates a conditioned response chain leading back to the initial conditioned response. He also suggests that the longer the sequence of sequents, the less likely it is that a victim will necessarily consciously associate them with their root. That is, the root can be far enough removed that a particular trauma response appears to be more directly affiliated with one or more recent sequents. This, explains Moore [25], is one reason why what he terms covert PTSD—symptoms related to an unrecognized or unremembered trauma—can be so difficult to treat. In the absence of addressing the root directly, there is always emotional charge available to be triggered. Pavlov established that there is a limit to the number of stimuli that can be associated, or "chained", by a dog. No such limit appears to exist in humans, however, a fact suggested by our use of language, itself a gigantic, organized, and highly sophisticated system of agreed-upon associations between words (stimuli) and concepts. Figure 2 represents a series of five incidents among a great many "sequents" that were experienced over a period of years by one person—a combat veteran. Each sequent is linked through association with a sixth "root" traumatic combat incident containing stimuli that included the sounds of children, the sound of a helicopter, and the loud noise of an explosion, as well as the sight of a tree line and the taste of chewing gum. Note that each succeeding sequent approaching the most recent (the one at the bottom of the figure) contains new stimuli in addition to others present in earlier incidents. Note too, however, that by the time the most recent incident occurs, the process of generalization through association has so broadened the range of effective stimuli or triggers that the theme or response—blinding rage—triggered by the original event, can now be triggered by other stimuli, *none* of which were present in the root incident.

When the victim repeatedly and in sequence reviews a series of incidents or experiences containing unpleasant symptoms, these sequents in effect collapse and the root incident becomes exposed [14]. As this occurs, the victim is allowed to inspect the experience; gain insight into the thoughts, sensations, and feelings suppressed in the original incident; and finally to reach an understanding of the traumatic experience(s) that is consistent with his/her perception of self and the world. With the relevant sequents addressed and the root incident eliminated, the victim can move into survivorship. If only some of the sequents are dealt with and the root incident remains intact, the victim may be unable to progress to survivorship, but may still experience significant relief [14].

Such victims (those experiencing significant relief) are akin to the walking wounded often referred to in history, stories, songs, and movies. They appear to not require immediate help and will even suggest they are okay. Yet emotionally, they are still a victim and, in spite of this victimization, they remain marginally or moderately functional. They consider themselves survivors because they have physically survived the traumatic event and the "victim" label is not consistent with how they perceive themselves. It would appear they are functional victims and are able to carry on for extended periods of time.

Although TIR is becoming best known as a treatment for psychological trauma, it can be used effectively in the treatment of specific irrational feelings, attitudes, and/or emotions [15]. TIR has several major strengths which suggest it is a good therapeutic technique. Primarily, as the reader will discover in later chapters of this book, the practice of TIR is intensely standardized. As Gerbode & Moore [15] suggest, this greatly reduces the influence

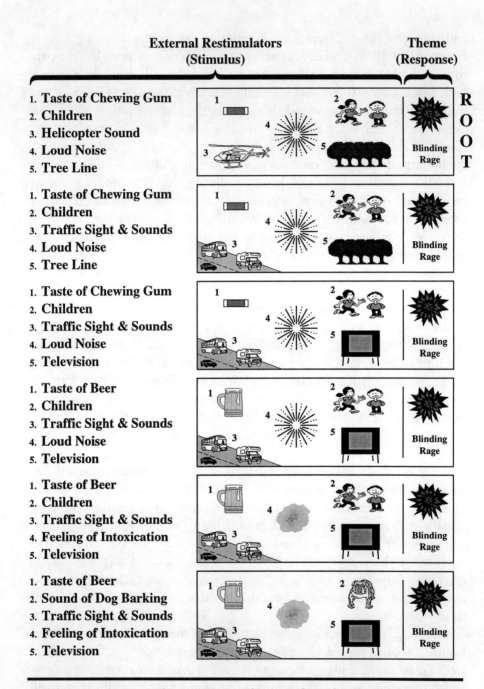

Figure 2 A sequence of traumatic incidents. (Adapted with permission from Ref. 14, p. 438.)

of the therapist's personality on the therapeutic outcome. As well, the TIR protocol effectively eliminates all the usual and expected therapeutic interventions. In fact, the therapist is referred to as a facilitator to remove the therapist's perceived identity as a psychopathologist. This suggests yet another strength of the approach: when the therapist's power to interpret, evaluate, or dispute is removed from the session, the responsibility for the success of the session becomes the client's, or viewer's, and this is enormously empowering.

TIR is one of a large number of procedures derivative of a subject called (after Freud) metapsychology. Those procedures have applications in the fields of both therapy and personal growth. The theory behind their development is beyond the scope of this book, but we have included a description and instructions for the use of one other metapsychological tool in addition to TIR. Called "Unblocking" [13a] (see Chapter 8 for a detailed exploration of this technique), it frequently serves as a very useful and effective compliment or adjunct to TIR. It is included in this book for that reason, and because it is relatively easy to learn and use.

TIR IN BROAD STROKES

2

During my initial TIR training in Menlo Park, I had someone in mind to start out with on my return to Idaho: a combat vet—Vietnam—who had been in the thick of a lot of killing and mayhem; a man who suffered the classic symptoms of Post Traumatic Stress Disorder, who "job-hopped" and who, frankly, I was tired of seeing show up in front of my desk on the average of once every four months, saying, "Lost my job again. I need another job. The family's getting hungry, and, oh, by the way, I've been drunk for the last three days ... and I'm broke." Well, that guy and I started down the road. Thinking back on it, I recall my thoughts as he relived his combat experiences. I can recall very distinctly.... Hmm! That's strange! I hadn't thought of it 'til now—that I was thinking, "That's not so bad; I did worse than that. I was in deeper crap than that. What's your problem, fella?"—those kinds of thoughts. I remembered Gerald's instructions, though: "Keep your mouth shut and let the system work". And I did.

That session was a long one, by the way, probably one of the longer ones that I've given. I may well have had an overrun or two, and mixed two or three incidents into the same string before it was all over, but it was dynamic at the end of it. I didn't miss the final end point. It blew in my face. It ... it was wonderful!

In the course of running down after the session was over, he mentioned that he had a friend that was in a town about thirty-five miles away—another Vietnam combat vet who was in a wheel chair. His story I've told before, but just real generally here, a fast one time through: "This fellow tried to commit suicide—the one in the wheel chair, that is. The first man I'd dealt with called me, and he and I went to the hospital. We talked, and the fellow was released the following day. I took him through a couple of sessions, and he went from suicidal to working full time in a coffee shop—and by the way, he's still there! He is the person who runs around in his chair and cheers everyone else up and says, "Hey! there is something about life...!" There's a guy who has now been working almost two years ... hadn't worked before that for five or six years ... had been under professional psychiatric care, medicated to the gills. Today, he is off medication and no longer under psychiatric care. My dealings with him lasted ... well ... over a period of about three months, we probably put in somewhere close to twenty hours of TIR. It was his decision to get off of the medications; it was his decision to quit psychiatric care; it was his decision to go back to work. Hey! Not too shabby, I would say offhand.

Guess we'd better take a short break.... [Tape pause.] Very interesting thing: I got a bit teary-eyed over that. It still brings joy to the heart.

TIR is a procedure intended to render benign the consequences of past traumatic events. Used correctly and in suitable circumstances, it eliminates virtually all of the symptoms of PTSD listed in the *DSM-IV* [1] and is capable of resolving a host of painful and unwanted feelings and emotions that have not surrendered to other interventions. According to Bisbey [4], TIR is an uncovering technique and has elements in common with other approaches that employ repetitive exposure and desensitization in mediating trauma, such as sequential analysis, direct therapeutic exposure, flooding, and implosion. It differs from each of them significantly, however, in a number of ways. For example, at no time during a TIR session does the protocol permit the therapist to offer any comments, interpretations, evaluations, disputations, or even validations to the client. Although tightly scripted, TIR provides a client-titrated exposure, and typically involves far more communication from the client than from the therapist. TIR leads, more often than not, to spontaneously client-generated insight, personal growth, and empowerment.

A vital part of the therapist's role in TIR consists of keeping the session and the client's attention tightly focused. The therapist always consults the client in deciding what to address in a given session and, once begun, each session continues until the presenting incident or target symptom (called a "theme") that the client and therapist have agreed to address in that session has been brought to an "end point" (see later discussion). At that point, the client will typically experience and voice, at a minimum, a sense of peace, respite, and relief. The client will no longer be haunted by the theme or incident and, in one way or another, the therapist will know that. On occasion, by the end of the session, the therapist will observe truly dramatic changes in the client's affect and ideation, manifest by laughter, expressions of joyous relief ("I can't *believe* I've suffered so long over that!") and the expression of major and life-changing cognitive shifts.

BASIC AND THEMATIC TIR

The first step of TIR is to identify the issue or "item"* that you are going to address. That might be your client's description of a "presented incident"—a specific incident, known and cited as troubling by the client—or a description of some content or theme that is common to a sequence of incidents experienced—a "thematic" item (see below). These two types of items—themes and presented incidents—are treated somewhat differently with TIR.

Basic TIR

If a known and severely traumatic incident or presented incident is readily accessible, it is usually a good idea to address it first, with the procedure called Basic TIR, before attempting to address thematic items. There may or may not turn out to be a sequence of earlier incidents underlying a presented incident, but the presented incident can often be handled as itself, without reference to earlier related material. Furthermore, having selected a specific incident in which your client is interested, you simply have the client go through it a number of times in his/her mind, reporting to you after each run-through what happened in the incident** and any thoughts or reactions he/she may have had at the time or while reviewing it. The client will generally experience great relief.

Thematic TIR

We have found it safe to assume that a high percentage of all negative feelings, attitudes, or undesirable impulses of which clients wish to rid themselves will, if pursued, be found to be *themes*: fear of men, the belief that women are not to be trusted, or a sudden rush of panic, for example. These themes,

---

* An *item* is a person, issue, question, topic, or incident that possibly or actually contains emotional charge and is accessible for handling by the client. Also, a word, phrase, or sentence that communicates such an entity.
** The client does not have to provide details of the incident.

feelings (e.g., fears), emotions, sensations, attitudes, beliefs,* and even some physical pains, in turn will be found to be contained in sequences of separate incidents, linked by the common theme(s) triggered, or restimulated, in them. Many of the incidents (*sequents*) in such sequences will be only secondarily traumatic—that is, traumatic not because they contain what Gerbode [14] has called primary pain, pain rooted in all but universally natural aversion, but only because they contain stimuli that have triggered earlier primary pain (see Figure 2). Such sequences will be found to culminate in *root* incidents that typically do contain primary pain—a real, or untriggered, independent source of trauma. Thoroughly viewing those root incidents will release the charge that has held in place the theme that linked the later incidents. Thus, although initially there may be no obvious connection between themes and the traumatic experiences that underlie them, Thematic TIR shows wide promise of being extremely effective in addressing and alleviating a wide variety of adjustment and anxiety disorders [8], bouts of depression, rage, panic attacks, phobias, and other painful and undesired conditions, all of which can be described or expressed as themes, and many of which turn out to have trauma as their source.

The facilitator handles a theme by asking the client to find an incident—any specific incident—in which that particular theme was present. If she is bothered by, say, "a feeling of not being able to stand men", you can ask her to recall a specific incident containing the feeling of not being able to stand men. You then take her through the incident several times until no further charge is released from it and you have reached an end point *or* until her attention moves, or can be redirected to an *earlier* incident containing the same theme, whereupon you address *that* one. The facilitator will eventually encounter a root incident, and at some point during the client's review of that incident, the client will experience, at a minimum, a feeling of relief, usually coupled with one or more realizations or insights. At that juncture, the end point, the facilitator stops running the theme.

END POINTS

Understanding the concept of an end point is critical to the successful use of TIR. If you do not grasp it, you will fail more often than not in your efforts to help people with the technique.

---

* Often akin to Ellis' "irrational Beliefs" (iBs), but *never,* in the case of TIR, identified as such by the therapist, let alone disputed.

There is an optimum time at which to end almost any activity or procedure, whether it be cooking pasta or addressing an issue or item with TIR.
At this end point, certain characteristic "indicators" appear. In the case of
pasta, one such indicator is that when it has been boiled just long enough,
a piece of it, when thrown, will stick to the wall of the kitchen.* However
determined, though, pasta has reached its end point when properly *al dente*.
It is not improved by being cooked longer.

When TIR has reached a proper end point, you will observe the following
indicators in the client:

- The client will feel—and manifest—relief from what was troubling.
- You will see the client relax and "lighten up" visibly.
- The client's attention will come out of the past and into the present.
- Often, the client will have some kind of significant insight.

*You must not stop TIR while your client is still feeling miserable or "locked into"
an incident!*

Obviously, then, as discussed elsewhere and required by the "Rules of
Facilitation" (see Chapter 5), flexible session lengths are essential to the
creation of the sort of safe environment required by TIR. It is important for
the facilitator to be able to continue a session until the client has reached an
end point, at which there are good feelings because something important has
been resolved. It is equally important for the facilitator to stop when such
an end point is reached. If the client feels confident that the facilitator will
give time to resolve anything encountered during a session, the client will
willingly get into highly charged areas. This is important, because a given
incident or thematic sequence may take anywhere from five minutes to two
or three hours to reach an end point. The average time is perhaps an hour
and a half, but this is highly variable.

Having said that, we borrow heavily from one of many invaluable
exchanges French and Gerbode have had with Steven Bisbey, in England over
the years of TIR's development. Some clients may in fact require more than
a single session to reach an end point. In such instances, some of the work
that goes into the attainment of true end points may take place between
sessions. That is one reason why it is a good idea to begin sessions by asking

---

* GDF swears by this particular indicator; others—his wife among them—prefer to rely on
somewhat less informal indicators. CJH likes alternately cooking and biting the pasta, waiting
for the white core to disappear.

the client whether, since the last session, the client has had any particular thoughts, feelings, or insights (s)he wishes to mention. Still, be careful not to violate the rule above: *do not stop TIR while the client is still feeling miserable or "locked into" an incident.* In an open-ended session, even if a full end point cannot be reached, the facilitator can almost always bring the client to a point at which any dramatic affect concerning the incident being run has subsided, and the client can "let it go," having no more interest in it at least for the time being. In doing so, the facilitator will have taken it to a "flat" point. In a subsequent session, then, the facilitator can and should always take up the incomplete procedure originally begun so as to fully complete it.

It may also bear mentioning that serious presenting incidents, although resolvable in and of themselves with TIR, do not occur in a vacuum. In some cases, more than TIR or more than one use or type of TIR will be required to resolve all of the subsidiary traumata that may have developed in the turbulent wake of a given incident. In the case of a rape, for example, there is potential for a myriad of events, phenomena, personnel, and issues to become associated with the precipitating event, one or more of which might be highly emotionally charged in a given instance and thus itself be in need of address as a separate issue. Such could be anything from the treatment the victim received in hospital or at the hands of the police, attorneys, or the media, to the reactions of intimates, to a fear of pregnancy or sexually trans-mitted diseases, to a court case, to men or sex in general, to existential issues: "Why me? What did I do to deserve that?" TIR, whether Basic or Thematic, would then, again, become only one of many possible "weapons" in the therapist's armamentarium. Although TIR might be the best procedure to use with a given client in addressing, say, a traumatic experience in court connected with the rape, it might very well not be the tool of choice with which to address, for example, the reactions of a particular intimate.

Again, when the TIR procedure has taken the requisite amount of emo-tional charge out of a traumatic incident or sequence, a certain set of phe-nomena will typically appear, indicating that the client has reached a valid end point:

- Positive indicators (PIs)*

---

* Positive indicators are those that suggest that an undesirable state is being or has been replaced by a desirable (or more desirable) one. PIs can and do include such manifestations in one's client as: expressions of relief, calm, or happiness; the onset of smiling or even laughter; often a change from present to past tense when referring to the theme or incident; as well as the elimination of negative affect earlier present in the session.

- Realization, insight, or expressed decision or intention
- Extroversion

These phenomena do not appear until the client has reached the root of a sequence and has reduced or eliminated the emotional charge contained within it. When such an end point occurs, it is important that the facilitator recognize the fact and stop working on that particular incident or sequence. It has now ceased to be part of the client's present. Furthermore, and this point cannot be overstressed, it is vitally important that the client feel confident that it has ceased to be a part of the *facilitator's* present as well, and that it will remain so forever unless for some reason the client should express a later interest in bringing it to the fore again. At the end point, the client reclaims the personal power that was tied up in maintaining the incident or sequence as part of the present. (S)he is no longer liable to having it triggered.*

During the session, as the client approaches an end point, the facilitator will generally observe that the client's indicators are improving and that the incident being run appears to be getting "lighter", or less painful. More often than not, the client will be visibly moving upward on the emotional scale as well (see Figure 3). Wait until the client has full positive indicators. Not infrequently, this will involve the client smiling or even laughing; at the least, the facilitator should observe expressions of relief, and indications that the client has attained a feeling of being at peace with the issue that has been addressed. Ideally, the client will express a realization, or mention a decision made at the time of the incident. This last shows that the client has contacted an aberrant intention or belief—one made or adopted at the time of the incident, since become inappropriate, and now unmade or forsworn. Such an expression is thus another good indicator of an end point.

If all of these signs are not yet present, the client may need to review the incident a few more times in order to reach a full end point. A good rule of thumb is: *Don't interrupt a client while (s)he is* [in the parlance of metapsychology] *"viewing" charged material.* If the client is still looking inward, it is not yet the time nor has the client reached the insight(s) needed in order to achieve a full end point. When the client reaches the end point, the cycle is complete and positive indicators will be manifested and demonstrated.

---

* (S)he may, however, still be somewhat affected if some of the same incidents are part of other, as yet undischarged, sequences. If so, you can reduce any remaining charge by running these other sequences.

EMOTION
EXHILARATION
ENTHUSIASM
CHEERFULNESS
CONSERVATISM
COMPLACENCY
AMBIVALENCE
ANTAGONISM
ANGER
RESENTMENT
COVERT HOSTILITY
ANXIETY
FEAR
GRIEF
APATHY

Figure 3   The Emotional Scale. (Reprinted with permission from Ref. 13, p. 30.)

Then the facilitator indicates to the client that the procedure is complete by saying something like, "OK, thanks. We'll stop with that."

When accompanied by positive indicators, the extroversion of your client's attention is the most reliable sign of an end point. Also, if the client says that the incident has no more charge on it, an adequate end point has been reached.

If the facilitator is unsure whether or not an incident is discharged, ask one or both of the following additional questions:

- How does the incident seem to you now?
- Did you make a decision at the time of the incident?

A positive answer to either of these questions, such as "It seems pretty uninteresting"... "Not much there anymore; I guess I just did what I

did"..."There's nothing more to it"... or "Well, yes, I think I decided that
_____"… will generally be accompanied by PIs and will then signal a valid
end point.

CHANGE AND THE EMOTIONAL SCALE

The various emotions that we experience in life can be arranged to form a
scale (see Figure 3, the Emotional Scale), in which the higher emotions are
more closely related to success and the lower ones are closer to failure. At
any given time, in general, or with respect to a specific activity in which we
are engaged, we occupy a certain point on that scale. Some people tend to
be enthusiastic much of the time; others to be characteristically angry, antag-
onistic, or bored (ambivalent). We may be generally cheerful, but anxious
about a sick child. Or anxious for the most part in the majority of our dealings
with life, but cheerful whenever we are playing golf or bridge.

In other words, the emotions that we feel are of two types: chronic and
acute. Depending on its nature, an emotion acts on us to provoke or inhibit
actions that will do either one of the following:

a. Promote the happiness and well-being of ourselves and those around
   us
b. Impair or frustrate the happiness and well-being of ourselves and
   those around us

As a rule, we tend to think of most emotions as being *acute*, that is, as
being caused by specific events in our lives and immediately responsive to
and reflective of those events. Someone sideswipes our car in a parking lot,
and we experience anger. We help a client, or win a game or a contract, and
feel elation, and so forth. Yet we all also tend to view life from the vantage
point of one or another *chronic* emotional state. By chronic, we mean more
or less stable, changing only momentarily as acute emotions gain dominance
for a time. We probably have all known someone whose chronic emotion
was anger, for example. Such a person's outlook on life tends to be characteristic, and many of his/her actions and responses are quite predictable: just
about everything we or anyone else does is *wrong* in his/her estimation, and
(s)he generally lets us know about it. (S)he is the first one to point out our
flaws, and the last to support a new idea, because (s)he knows it is a bad one:
"Yeah, *sure!*," such a person will say, "but what about _____?! It never

worked before and it sure as hell won't *now!*" In general, such people are inclined to try to stop or *impede* things, both people and activities.

Any one of the levels outlined in the Emotional Scale can be either acute or chronic. Whichever it is, it colors the world that is seen and lived in by the person experiencing the emotion. When chronic, in fact, it tends actually to *structure*, to dictate the form of, the world one lives in, acting as a self-fulfilling prophesy. In facilitating TIR, the therapist will be concerned with the client's chronic *and* acute emotions. The first will dictate the overall case plan, the strategy, as it were; the second, the facilitator's immediate actions, the tactics at any given moment in a session. The client's chronic emotion will tell a great deal about how the client views life and other people. It will also tell the kind of world the client experiences living in, and the kind of people and events that populate and characterize that world. The chronic emotion of a PTSD case will generally be well into the bottom half of the scale (at or below antagonism). Our goal as facilitators is to allow that to *change*, and to the degree that the facilitation is successful, it will do so. Three things will happen, and both the facilitator and the client will be able to see them clearly:

1. The chronic emotion will gradually become significantly higher and more stable on the scale than it was before TIR began;
2. The client will start to enjoy life a great deal more; and
3. The world around the client will seem to change for the better...and in fact it will do so.

THE STEPS OF TIR

As we have earlier noted, TIR can be explained in terms of a number of different models, including psychoanalysis, client-centered therapy, Pavlov [25], and exposure-based work. Certainly TIR has aspects in common with each of them. The elements of TIR that perhaps differentiate it most clearly from any of its predecessors are:

- Its very strict protocol, the boundaries of which are sharply delineated by what we call the Rules of Facilitation (see Chapter 5).
- The particular way in which we train therapists to handle the communication that takes place in a session (see Chapters 3 and 4).

The most spare and elegant form of TIR—and the one you will use most often when working with traumatized clients—we call Basic TIR.* In brief, it consists of the following steps:**

1. *Consulting your client's interest, you select an incident to "run", or address.* Of course, in almost any case presenting with—and because of—a known, single-incident trauma such as a rape or a plane crash, this assessment is essentially done before you have begun, and the presenting incident is the one you will be running with your client.

2. *Find out where the incident happened.* You may get responses such as, "It was when we lived in Virginia", "It happened at Mom's house", "I was on the redeye flight from California", or "We were at Uncle Jack's farm". Any response indicating a place is acceptable.

3. *Find out how long the incident lasted.**** Responses such as, "It lasted for fifteen minutes", "I was in it for over an hour", "We were only there for a few moments", or "It was just long enough for me to smoke a cigarette" would all be acceptable.

4. *Have your client focus on the* moment *the incident occurred.* You are asking your client to prepare for the TIR viewing by putting attention on the beginning of the incident.

5. *Have your client close his/her eyes (if it is comfortable to do so).* Closing eyes often helps the viewer "see" the incident more clearly by removing the distractions of the environment.

6. *Ask your client to describe the scene at the moment when the incident began.* This begins the description of the incident but it is only the beginning moment (to set the stage, so to speak).

7. *Have your client silently (re)"view" the incident from beginning to end.* Before your client begins to tell what happened, (s)he must put it into a perspective. This silent viewing helps.

8. *Have the client tell you what happened.* Your client's answer to this instruction may be a spare outline, or it may be very detailed.

9. *Repeat steps 4, 7, and 8.*

---

* Here and in all our discussions of protocol, we assume that some suitable form of screening has earlier taken place, and that the therapist has determined that TIR is an appropriate tool to use with the client in question. See Chapter 10.
** We describe the protocol in detail in Chapter 5.
*** If the client is using an event that has a long history (e.g., physical abuse over years), you will want the client to focus on just one of the incidents.

From this point, you facilitate the viewing by having the client repeat the cycle of going to the start of the incident, moving through it silently to the end, and then telling you what happened (steps 4, 7, and 8) until the client reaches an end point. However, there are conditions that will prohibit an end point; they are detailed in Chapter 6.

The principal difference between Basic and Thematic TIR has little to do with the questions and instructions you will give your client. Those remain essentially the same. Rather, it has to do with timing and sequence, and we address those and other points of protocol elsewhere.

MANAGING COMMUNICATION IN VIEWING

3

The first combat vet: we took him through, oh, about twenty five hours by the time that he felt that he was through. We found that most all of what he had hung his combat experiences on went a little bit deeper than that—many times back to, oh, age four or five ... in there, though he was not specific. That fellow is still working, still with the same job that he obtained within thirty days of completing TIR.

And while the thought crosses my mind: when I arrived at Job Service in Lewiston, Idaho, back in April of 1985, there were in excess of 150 disabled veterans on the rolls, seeking employment. I worked with those people up until the time that I went to California to receive my TIR training, and so we had close to five years that I worked very hard with those folks to put 'em to work and keep 'em in jobs. I would say at the time that I went to California, I still had a hundred and twenty of those people on the roles, seeking employment. With the skills learned through TIR training (and I'm talking the one-week, forty hour intensive course that Gerald gave me and Lori Beth) I would estimate that I have worked with close to sixty of those people, anywhere from two hours to twenty hours, max, the average probably running closer to 14 or 15 hours. And out of those 60 people that I worked with on TIR, I had two—that's one, two!—left on the roles, seeking employment, when I left Idaho for Germany three weeks ago.

I have had failures. Every one of my failures has been exactly where Gerald told me it would occur—in a place where the mind was not available: mind-altering drugs ... alcohol. Those are the two main causes. Mind not available

> *... I am not capable of getting through with TIR.... Hey, that's alright. I basically ceased working with those types of people, merely telling them that it's their choice, that once they get to the point—and they can do whatever they want to—I will be available, if I'm geographically in the area, to assist once they're clean. Those failures, a total of four, I had to find out for myself. So be it. I did.*

As we have earlier suggested, TIR and most of the other procedures that have come out of the study of metapsychology [14], including Unblocking (see Chapter 8), derive a major part of their efficacy not only from their simplicity, but also from the fact that they are administered according to protocols that involve considerably more than the actual (and basically rote) procedures themselves. Underlying the application of all metapsychology procedures are two principal *substrata*. The first has to do with the facilitator's control of the *communication* that takes place in a session; the second, with his/her adherence to a body of laws called the Rules of Facilitation. This chapter addresses the facilitator's handling of communication.

The TIR procedure itself is forgiving, up to a point, and its very roteness makes it easy to become competent in its use, providing that the facilitator assigns sufficient importance to the materials covered in this chapter and the two that follow.

If you observe the rules and principles covered here, the TIR procedure will generally work well, and you will be successful. But note that these data, when taken as a whole, represent highly significant departures from what you would normally expect to find in either conventional therapies or even garden-variety quotidian communication. In fact, as you will see, they will sometimes require that you act, or *refrain* from acting, in ways that may at first seem artificial or unnatural to you. But you will soon see for yourself just how helpful and powerful those tools are. And if you fail to operate with them as guidelines, you *can* fail with TIR quite easily.*

Much of the skill required of a facilitator has nothing to do with his/her knowledge of the theory or technique of TIR. Rather, it lies in expertly managing communication in the session while adhering strictly to the Rules of Facilitation (discussed in Chapter 5). These skills enable you to create a suitable and *safe space* in which viewing can take place.

---

* The admonitions in this introduction above cannot be overstressed. Had there been a way of presenting them here in neon lights, we would have done so.

A SAFE SPACE

We assume it to go without saying that neither you nor any other part of the environment will actually be *attacking* your client during the session. So why do we stress the term, *a safe space*, and what exactly do we mean by it?

We emphasize it because only within the confines of a truly safe space do we ever really take down our "antennae" and turn our mental and emotional "radar" *off*, rather than merely reducing its sensitivity. In other words, we are attempting to describe the creation of a level of perceived safety that significantly exceeds what we generally think of as "safe". By safe, we mean that your client is able to determine* far more of what (s)he is going to receive from the session with you, the only other person in the environment, than if (s)he were present at, say, a perfectly safe dinner party or simply talking with a friend.

Consider the following: in almost any such situation, although we may feel perfectly safe in the normal sense of the word, our "radar" is still generally at least on "standby", not truly off. Our attention is still being pulled *outward*, if only by the need or desire to be aware of our friend, or the conversation of others, or simply to avoid bumping into the furniture. This is the case when the space is conventionally safe. As it becomes slightly less so—when, for example, "politics" enters into the picture (our friend may be after the job we are hoping for, or it's a staff party)—our radar "sweep" begins in earnest, and our attention becomes more and more fixed on the environment and the intentions of others sharing it, and less and less available to focus on anything out of the immediate present environs. Successful viewing, how-ever, involves intense concentration on material that is often elusive or dif-ficult to confront. It requires, in fact, that the viewer's full attention be available for him/her to focus on items, incidents, and considerations that are not part of the present. So even a small degree of "un-safety" is counter-productive.

Because of this, the way a facilitator handles the communication in a session is extremely important, so much so that over the course of teaching a four-day TIR workshop, we spend at least a full day with the participants working as dyads, practicing a series of exercises designed to break communication

---

* The degree of confidence we have in our ability to make accurate determinations is what helps us resolve whether or not we feel safe in a given setting. To the degree that we can predict a nonthreatening future *and have confidence in that prediction*, we feel truly safe. It is the absence of such confidence that makes the environment feel less than perfectly safe, and thus demanding of our attention to one degree or another.

down into its individual components. The mastery of such a skill is the difference between a facilitator who will get acceptable results when things are going "by the book", and one who can use communication to create the additional margin of safety we have previously described. Such a facilitator will achieve excellent outcomes even when matters have gone awry at one or another point over the course of a session.* In the following discussion of communication, we present not the communication exercises themselves, but a summary of their key elements. The importance of this material on communication and its relevance to the effective use of TIR is suggested by the following comments, excerpted from a chapter written by Dr. Wendy Coughlin for an as-yet unpublished book on the clinical use of TIR (reprinted here with her permission):

> TIR provides a paradigm for accessing traumatic material through the client's associational pattern without directing the content. The basic workshop in TIR challenged the very tenets of my earlier training. In many of us, years of training and experience in assessing the organizational patterns of human thought and family systems evolve into a stance of "therapist as sage". In retrospect, I saw that I delighted in showing off my agility in deciphering human behavior and emotions. A fair degree of accuracy can be achieved by this method, but it leaves you defenseless when emotions are based on idiosyncratic, unconscious associations. It was clear I could not influence my clients' investigation of their own cognitive material and expect to uncover those most critical and individualistic associations.

> Fortunately, the TIR method recognizes the need to "untrain" a natural tendency to encourage and reinforce while listening to a client. The Communication Exercises (CEs) focus on training the participant to maintain a truly neutral posture. This neutrality directly opposes most therapeutic techniques which include many subliminal approvals and encouragement (verbal as well as nonverbal). Handling communication in a session, as the exercises dispose one to do, disrupts most conditioned responses to client statements. It clearly and comprehensively reveals flaws in therapeutic postures designed to be "unconditional" and informs participants of alternate ways of responding. How strange that those who train others in *nondirective* processes frequently fail to address the subtle encouragement offered by a nod or a well-placed 'uh-humm'.

---

* In fact, you will find that the skills learned through these exercises will be enormously helpful not only in communicating with clients in session but in all the communicating you do in your life.

The principals of learning theory evidence the strength of these often subtle reinforcers. Earlier, before taking the TIR training, we had considered them to be potentially destructive to the therapeutic process. Responses frequently mask meaning by diverting the viewer in the direction of the facilitator's interest. The communication exercises assure the therapist's close evaluation of all levels of communication. The terminology used to identify therapist and client also reflects the way that communication is managed in a TIR session, and signals another departure from traditional, clinical training. The therapist becomes a *facilitator* and the client/patient, a *viewer*. This appropriate divergence of terminology from mainstream psychology acknowledges the actual function of the "therapist" and the "client" in a TIR session. The therapist does not *provide* therapy but rather *facilitates*; the client is not a *patient being treated* but a *viewer developing awareness*. The viewer is an active participant investigating his/her own experience. The facilitator's function is to guide the process, not the content, and to be interest*ed* rather than interest*ing*.

We break communication down into eight parts, or aspects, each "nesting" in, or built upon, the ones preceding it. The communication exercises referred to above address each of those parts in turn. The discussion that follows will not directly address every one of them. Rather, our intention will be to describe the requirements concerning the handling of communication which, if not met by the therapist in a TIR or other metapsychologically oriented session, will greatly reduce the likelihood of attaining full end points. The exercises, in sequence, involve:

1. Being Present
2. Interest
3. Maintaining Interest
4. Delivery
5. Acknowledgment
6. Getting Questions Answered
7. Handling Concerns and Originations

BEING PRESENT

What we mean by "being present" is essentially the same thing Babba Ram Das [9] meant when he wrote about *being here now*, it is being wherever one *is*, comfortably *there*, with one's attention in the present place and moment *and nowhere else.* Gautama Sidhartha referred to *mindfulness.* It is being there without wondering when we will have a chance to get a word in edgewise, or trying to remember if we left the freezer door ajar, or thinking about the good impression we are (or may not be) making on the person in front of us, or the wisdom we are (or are not) imparting. To the degree that we are really being present with a client or anyone else, we will be simply aware, and receptive, and the person with whom we are being present will feel that "presence". Being present is the first requisite to truly good communication, and anyone wishing to facilitate TIR will find that practice in being unremittingly present will serve them well in sessions, which, in TIR, can sometimes go on for a considerably longer period of time than the conventional 50 minutes. In workshops, we practice this briefly in an exercise that consists of sitting face to face with another person with one's eyes closed and one's attention focused on one's perceptions of the present moment.*

INTEREST

Interest** is the next requirement in effective communication. We define interest as "directed attention", a definition that represents an effort on our part to place interest under the conscious control of the person who is experiencing it, because (a) it *can* be so placed and (b) it *should* be.

Life conspires to make it easy not to realize that we can and do truly have control over our own interest; there are so many "interesting" things and people out there, and so many "uninteresting" ones as well. The quality of interest—or more accurately, perhaps, of "interesting-ness"—seems always to be contained in the object of interest, in the *thing* we are interested in.

And it is certainly true that our interest can be attracted by something we find "interesting", or repelled by something or someone "boring" or "uninteresting". The adjectives describe the thing, after all; they tell us that this one is interesting—that it "contains interest"—and that that one is not. A man sees an attractive woman and, at her feet on the sidewalk, a dead leaf. He

---

* We do this with closed eyes because to open one's eyes adds a new and significant element to the exercise. See the next section.
** We have not always called this facet of communication *interest*, although interest has always been a key aspect of the exercise we do in workshops to teach this. Because the exercise involves participants facing each other in pairs and looking directly at each other, we have in the past called it *confronting.* We changed it to *interest* for the same reason that the Bisbeys have elected to call it *contact.* "Confront" carries a connotation of antagonism, something definitely not a part of what we are trying to describe.

will very likely find the woman interesting and the leaf not so, *unless,* perhaps, he chances to be a gay botanist, in which case he may find the opposite to be the case. What are we describing here? We think of it loosely as "interest", but it really is *attention;* if our attention is attracted to something, we say, by definition, that that thing is "interesting".

So where does this quality, this entity, interest, actually reside, and who is—or should properly be—in control of it? Interest is the word we use to describe the phenomenon of attention that seems to have been attracted by the object of interest. We use it typically to describe our uncontrolled attention when the latter is directed to and seemingly "pulled out of" us by some element in our environment. But look again at the definition of interest that we offered at the beginning of this discussion: "directed attention". Note that we have not specified by what or whom the attention was to be directed.

In fact, interest resides in the person feeling it. If you wish to, you can consciously create and maintain your own interest in anything (or anyone), with or without any external cause. Reread the definition and you will perhaps see how, when you deliberately and intentionally* direct your attention to another person, you find that you have become interested in him/her, and both of you will immediately experience a powerful positive effect on the quality of your communication.

If we wish truly to create and maintain interest in another person, we need to be able to be with him/her *comfortably.* The Rogerian concept of *unconditional positive regard,* very much a requirement of the successful facilitation of TIR, requires at a minimum that we be able to maintain interest in virtually anything our client may present to us—with equanimity, and without the necessity to react. A physical flinch is not the only kind of flinch there is. It is possible to "flinch" mentally or emotionally as well, and all too often, if we permit it, it can happen in a session when we are dealing with a traumatized client. We *sympathize* with our client, and our attention goes to an image of how horrible *we* would feel if the loss he/she is describing had happened to *us.* Or perhaps something similar *has* happened to us, and we

---

* The word *intention* is deserving of some attention itself. In normal parlance, we use it to mean something only somewhat more under our control than a fairly vague *wish:* "I *intended* to get here at six, but got held up in traffic." There is another sort of intention, however, and that is the one we mean here; it is one that truly brooks no other outcome than the one we intend. When we decide to stand up, for example, barring restraint or physical disability, we simply stand up. It happens. We don't *wonder* if it will happen or imagine that it might not. Experientially, we simply know it will because we intended it to. That second sort of intention is the one to which we are referring here.

try our best to suppress the triggering that occurs as our client talks. We would maintain that clients *read* that sort of thing in us—they *feel* our discomfort, much as we do. They may never articulate the feeling, but it will be there, and to whatever degree that it is, we have made the space *unsafe* for them, in the sense that their attention to one degree or another will have left their own story and gone onto us and our reaction to it—our "flinch".

A good definition of *flinch* is "a sudden, uncontrolled cessation of interest in a trigger". And a flinch can be as minute and subtle as a tiny shiver on a warm day or as blatant as a full-blown dramatization of a flashback to combat. In each case, and always to some degree unconsciously, attention has left the trigger in the present and gone to the entity in the past that has been stimulated by the trigger.

TIR requires of you as a facilitator the ability to face and look directly at a client without flinching—either overtly or covertly, as above—or avoidance. In other words, with interest. When we teach interest in a workshop, we talk about and try to model simply being fully *aware* of the person in front of us, consciously paying attention to them with the *intention* of doing so, being present comfortably with them, and not necessarily having to *do* anything with or about them at all.

Genuinely and simply being interested in another person is that part of communication with which people generally seem to have the most difficulty. We have workshop participants practice this skill by simply facing and look-ing directly at another person while seated comfortably. Like meditation, this can be done as an exercise to good effect for quite a considerable length of time. It differs from meditation perhaps only in the sense that the object of meditation is the person in front of you—not a common focus of medita-tion—and because rather than thinking about (or meditating upon) that person, we work to simply be aware of him/her as (s)he *is*, in the *present*.

We probably have all had, at some point, the experience of talking to someone who is not really interested in us. Such a person manifests a lack of interest in various ways, such as a glassy stare, a bored or vacant look, shifting eyes. On the other hand, someone who is interested in you appears alive and focused. When someone looks at you, that someone *sees you*. You do not get the feeling that the attention has gone elsewhere. Such a person can put attention where (s)he wants it to be and can keep it there as long as (s)he wishes. Such a person does not easily get distracted or caught up in his/her own thoughts. The attention, rather, is directed *outward*, toward the environment and the world around—in a session, toward the cli-ent—and not constantly turned *inward* on one's own thoughts, feelings, and considerations. When we deal with such a person, we feel as if we really are in contact with him/her, as if we are connected. By the same token, when someone who purports to be communicating with us isn't truly interested in us, we feel *dis*connected, and our level of trust goes down, slowly or precipitously, depending on our own level of awareness.

In talking about interest, we are talking about awareness: consciousness, the ability and willingness to perceive. A "higher state of consciousness" or "increased awareness" involves at the very least an enhanced ability to create and maintain interest, to really *notice*.

When we have trouble being interested in another person, we tend to interpose something between ourselves and the other, and then to confront "by way of" that thing, whatever it is. It could be our posture, expression, or body language—arms crossed over our chest, or a tolerant, avuncular smile, for instance. It could also be a displacement activity, such as sipping coffee or scribbling lengthy notes. Not uncommonly, it is an attitude that we are manifesting, or some identity or role that we are more or less unconsciously being, or playing, instead of just being there and being interested as ourselves.

In TIR and Unblocking sessions, it is extremely important that your full attention be on your viewer. Most mistakes made in administering either of the procedures stem directly from the facilitator's interest—direct attention—wandering just long enough to miss the proper end point of the session, or for a negative indicator to flit briefly across the client's face, unnoticed and unhandled; hence the importance of our paying very close attention to this aspect of communication and, in workshops, to an exercise designed to provide practice in creating interest at will and thus in preventing such lapses from happening.

INTEREST*ED* VS. INTEREST*ING*

Most of us have been *programmed* virtually from birth to be interest*ing*, or to attract attention. It goes against the grain to simply be interest*ed*, to observe and listen carefully to another person without having to do or say anything. But the degree to which we are able to do just that is the degree to which we will be able confidently to address and resolve the issues that TIR is capable of resolving, even while under stress of the sort that one frequently encounters in running TIR with heavily traumatized clients. The more interest*ing* we are to our client, the more of our client's attention we attract during a session of TIR—as, for example, by passing a box of tissues or offering sympathetic interjections—the more certain it is that the session will be a rough and unproductive one, and the more likely that the theme or incident we are attempting to address will remain to one degree or another emotionally charged and unresolved at the end of it.*

DELIVERY

Simply put, delivery is that part of communication that has to do with how spoken words are *delivered* by one person to another. It involves volume and tone of voice, pacing, accent, and the interest and intention of the speaker. In a TIR session, you want your words, interest, and intention *and nothing else* to *get across* to your client. Again, the reason for this has to do with where your client's attention needs to be if (s)he is going to run TIR successfully: if you speak too loudly or too softly, if your tone of voice is distracting in any way,** if you speak too quickly or too slowly or in any way that causes your client to need or want to put her attention on *you* rather than on your question, instruction, or acknowledgment, then the session will go less quickly and smoothly than it should.

Another point concerning delivery that bears particularly on your administration of TIR and Unblocking: because both of these procedures are tightly scripted and require of you the seemingly unnatural action of repeating *verbatim* something you have already said, often many times in a row, it is vital that you be able to do so without *sounding* as if you are. The more interest you are able to put into whatever question you are asking or instruction you give, the less likely it is that you will get something from your client other than a response appropriate to what you have asked him/her. And you will find that it is possible to generate interest anew in a session each time

---

* As Rachel Naomi Ramen has observed, "A loving silence often has far more power to heal …than the most well-intentioned words" (R. N. Ramen, M.D., *Kitchen Table Wisdom: Stories That Heal,* Putnam Publishing, New York, 1996, p. 144.)

** On occasion, we have had students who acquired over their years of training and experience as therapists a sort of "bedside manner" that crept into their voices as soon as they began to practice any kind of co-facilitation in the workshop. In normal conversation, it wasn't there, and they simply sounded like themselves. In brief, when they were "theraping", they were "being a therapist" instead of being natural (being themselves), and when that happens, it sounds artificial. A client's attention will often be drawn to such a therapist, and because (s)he sounds *unreal* to the client, it will put a distance between the two, although the client will doubtless never mention it. Almost invariably, when we have indicated that phenomenon to such a participant in a workshop, (s)he has been able to recognize it.

you ask a question, even if you are asking the same question repeatedly. Each time you ask the question, you need to ask it as though it had never occurred to you to ask that question before.

Your asking a question, the client's answer, and your acknowledgment of the answer, taken together constitute a cycle and, as such, define a period of time. Repeating the question without variation in a new period of time does *not* mean that you should attempt to replicate in a robotic manner the same tone or inflection, question after question. It does mean that you ask the original question anew, as if you had never asked it before, without varying the wording of the question at all. Do not make every question sound exactly like the last one, but do not make a conscious effort to deliberately vary the tone each time you ask it either. Each time you ask the question, start a new communication cycle, with new interest and in a new period of time in which you must receive an answer and acknowledge the answer. If you aren't able to put *new interest** into everything you say in TIR and Unblocking (it is possible to do just that, with practice) your viewer will quickly get the idea that you are bored or unhappy with him/her and you will "lose" the client. You will not know why, and (s)he may not be able to state why, but it will happen anyway. If TIR is to work as it should, your client must feel that your communication really comes from *you*—a live, interested person—and not from a book, or from some artificial identity you have created.

Finally, although in everyday life we naturally use body movements and gestures to express ourselves, it is important not to do so thoughtlessly in a TIR session because they can attract the attention of your viewer. Their complete absence could well be a distraction, too however: if your client thinks that (s)he is dealing with a robot, you will also lose him/her, of course! In summation, what is important is not that you communicate without any facial expression or body motions, but that you be *able* to at will, as appropriate.

ACKNOWLEDGMENT

The TIR and unblocking procedures consist of a myriad of separate and discrete cycles of communication, most consisting of a question or instruction from you, the facilitator, followed by a response from your viewer, followed in turn by an acknowledgment from you. You, the facilitator, must

---

* Recall our statement that each of these parts of communication includes within it, and/or relies upon, the ones that precede it.

assume responsibility for acknowledging—and thus for closing off, or *ending*—each one of these cycles in such a way that your client knows (s)he has been heard and understood, and can "let go of" that particular piece of communication. It is really rather as if every time you (1) ask your client a question or give him/her an instruction and (2) (s)he answers or complies and (3) *you acknowledge the answer*, you have established a boundary between yourself and the subject of the client's communication. The question or instruction you give your client is a box, the answer or compliance is the contents, and your acknowledgment is the knot tied in the string around the box that keeps it from flying open again; properly given, your acknowledgment really does have the potential to allow your viewer to "put it away" or "let it go" forever—*whatever* "it" is.

"Why are you going on about this?", you may be thinking. "I don't need to be told to acknowledge my clients!" But do you simply *acknowledge* them? Or are you possibly inclined to do something else as well, something *more*? Most of us are.

As therapists, most of us are inclined (indeed, have been *trained)* to use subtly evaluative statements or comments or partial acknowledgments* rather than simple, clean, full, *unencumbered* acknowledgments of the sort we are attempting to describe and espouse here for use with TIR—plain, vanilla-flavored *acknowledgments!*

Such as what? Well, such as: "OK", or "Thanks", or "I got that", or "All right". There can be no rote form of acknowledgment, of course, although "All right" is more than adequate in a very large percentage of instances during a viewing session. "Good", and "Fine" are acceptable; even "Gotcha" or "Thank you very much", depending entirely on the client and the context and the tone of voice in which they are uttered. "I see" and "I understand" are both very risky in certain situations. For example, a combat veteran or rape victim may not take kindly to hearing "I understand" from a therapist that (s)he knows is not one; and therefore, could not *possibly* understand. And if you happen to be that therapist and your client does not choose to let you know that (s)he has decided you're "just another damned shrink", you will have lost the ability to help him/her–(s)he will have written you off.

Comments such as "You have every right to feel that way" are not acknowledgments at all. They may well have a place somewhere, but we have found them to have none in the administration of TIR in its most effective form,

---

* See Coughlin's observations presented previously in this chapter, and the example that follows.

because it is far too strong an invitation to the client to put attention on the therapist and the therapist's opinion. In the purely person-centered viewpoint from which TIR must be administered, it is up to the *client* and not the therapist to determine what the client has or has not the right to feel.

Consider the following: our female client says, sobbing, "God ... I wish I didn't, but I *hate* that bastard for what he forced me to do!", and out of a perfectly valid wish to be helpful and supportive, we say something like, "You have every right to feel that way." We say that because we want to normalize a phenomenon for our client, to let her know that it is all right and permissible to have and express feelings. And of course it *is*. But such a response is *not* a simple acknowledgment. A simple acknowledgment would let the client know only what we want her to know: that she has been heard with interest. But a remark about her "right" does more than that. It is evaluative. It does not simply acknowledge the client's expression and close that particular "box" for that time. As a communication, it really does not do *only* what we intended it to. It does not *just* say to the client, in effect, "OK, I got that, and it's OK to feel that wa*y or any other way you may decide you want to feel* and to express it." Instead, our comment is open to being perceived by the client as a *judgment*—ours, and not the client's—concerning what feelings it is permissible or even *right* for our client to have and express. This example is too much like saying to her, "It's *right* to feel hate in that situation". And maybe it is! But just maybe, from some happier viewpoint at which our client, given the freedom to do so, may arrive upon further reflection, it *isn't*!

What would happen if, instead of normalizing, we left her to her own devices and simply directed her to look at and describe events and her thoughts about them at her own pace, evaluating them for herself, and reaching conclusions that she can feel quite free to reevaluate and *drop* if a second look—or a third, or a *tenth!*—enables her to reach one that suits her better and makes her happier? Perhaps, all by herself, our client would arrive at a self-empowering, life-changing realization concerning, say, the damage *she* realized she was doing to herself by clinging to a hatred or resentment that she *didn't* have to feel. She might find a relief in forgiveness that far exceeds the relief she earlier felt in expressing her hatred.

At that point she might drop the hate like an old glove, secure in the comfortable knowledge that we, the authority, *had nothing invested in any other denouement.* But if earlier, rather than simply acknowledging it, we have made evaluative comments suggesting that our client's less-examined and conflicting viewpoint was a *valid* one, what then?

Then, however inadvertently, we have lent the weight of our authority to a viewpoint that she may come to feel is one she no longer wishes to hold: "You know, I *don't* have the right to feel that way! I've been giving myself that right and I'm going to stop it! It's been wrecking my life, and it's unnecessary! I haven't been hurting *him*; more to the point, I've been hurting *myself!*" But to make such a change, she must now deal with the fact that we, the *authority*, have already suggested to her that her earlier, less examined, and conflicting viewpoint was the *correct* one: "You *do* have every right to feel that way".

She is engaged in peeling an onion, as it were. At one layer, she has perhaps blamed herself for events in no way her responsibility; at another, deeper one, she has found and finally expressed the raging hatred for the perpetrator that she'd suppressed for years and perhaps had never before admitted to herself, let alone to anyone else; at a deeper layer yet, she discovers the power of forgiveness. Both discoveries represent real progress, but any attention beyond simple acknowledgment that *we* as her facilitator focus on the first will significantly reduce the likelihood of her making the second, deeper one, certainly as quickly as she might—which is to say, within the space of that same session. By simply acknowledging each layer of the onion as she describes it to us, instead of interpreting, disputing, *or* validating it, we make it possible for her to simply put it aside—if *she* feels there may be more to discover—and to continue to move closer to the core of her own reality *by herself.*

And that is an enormously empowering experience for the client, albeit a somewhat humbling one for the therapist, for we discover that the client doesn't need nearly as much of our wise counsel as we may have thought she did. But if we are willing thus to fade into the background during a session, to relinquish our omniscience, our need to comment, to intercede, or interweave—to "help", in short—we will often receive enormous rewards; certainly you will find this to be true in your use of TIR and related techniques. In the words of one therapist, "I learned from experience that no matter what pearls of wisdom I imparted in a therapy session, they didn't have the positive impact that the client's *own* realizations had. Furthermore, I found that when I did nothing but acknowledge and direct the client's attention, the impact was even more profound. The client would sort it out for himself. And this is empowering" [4a].

By evaluating rather than simply acknowledging any position that our client takes in the course of examining his/her past and his/her thoughts about it, we either force him/her to defend it (if our evaluation has been negative), or force him/her later to feel (s)he must dispute us if (s)he comes to see a reason to *change* it. In either case, we have unwittingly made cognitive shifts much more difficult for the client to experience than (s)he could or should have been.

The proof of this, of course, is in the pudding. Clients who have gone through TIR generally reach end points at which they have resolved the theme or incident they set out to resolve, and when asked to evaluate the experience, they typically express great appreciation for having been permitted to change their ideas and perceptions fluidly without comment or evaluation from their facilitator.

Acknowledgment is not an unimportant or inconsequential part of communication. It is vital. Its power for both good and bad is enormous, and although we pay lip service to it, that power is generally unrecognized. Yet poor or nonexistent acknowledgments have doubtless acted as triggers that have led to *murder,** albeit infrequently, let alone to the creation of simple irritation, unsafe spaces, and failed therapy. Common errors include situations where an acknowledgment:

- Is absent
- Does not convey the impression that we have understood what the speaker said
- Is too soft or too loud
- Is delayed or premature
- Sounds unnatural or violates some other aspect of good "delivery"
- Does not fully complete the cycle of communication, so that the speaker feels that (s)he is expected to continue speaking, to say something else
- Is overwhelming
- Contains some sort of overt or covert comment, interpretation, or evaluation**
- Is overly long or elaborate

Note that acknowledgment does not have to denote agreement *or* disagreement, nor should it, in a TIR or Unblocking session. It simply means "Thank you ... I've heard you ... I've got what you've said ... I'm interested." A full acknowledgment *stops* your client's communication; it *controls* it.

---

* Examined in context, statements such as: "You never listen to me" "I really don't matter to you at all, do I?" and "You don't care about me and you never have!" will be found to have been usually preceded—at a minimum—by numerous undelivered acknowledgments.
** This could be nothing more than a raised eyebrow or the slightest hint of a dubious frown.

It is worth taking a moment to look at the idea of control. The word "control" itself is potentially loaded for many of us because our thoughts about it are so frequently accompanied not by pictures of control, but by images of what happens all too often when things have gone *out* of control (e.g., a child being spanked, or police with batons beating protesters). In fact, control in and of itself is never bad. It consists of nothing more, really, than three things. To control something, anything—a car, a thought, a project, or a cycle of communication in a therapeutic setting—we need to be able to get it started, or moving, to keep it moving as long as we wish it to, and then to stop it. As facilitators of TIR, we use a *question* or *instruction* to start our client's communication or activity (such as introspection, or viewing), our *interest* to keep it going, and our *acknowledgment* to stop it. Acknowledgment is, then, simply the final step of controlling your client's communication.

And from your client's viewpoint, properly done, such control does *not* feel like being beaten with a baton! Rather, it feels like a seatbelt on a winding mountain road. It feels safe, comfortable, and secure, and not unpleasantly constricting in the least. On the contrary, its absence is missed.

Note also that *timing* is essential in giving an acknowledgment. If your acknowledgment is too quick, your client will feel pressured, or will feel that you have not taken the time to really understand him/her. On the other hand, if your acknowledgment is too long in coming, your client will feel that you are preoccupied and not really interested.

Here again is another of those instances in which you can see the "nesting" of these aspects of communication, one within the next. Interest, discussed earlier, plays a large part in acknowledgment—if you have maintained genuine interest in what your client is saying to you or doing in response to an instruction, you will find that your acknowledgments will be both effective and effortless.

Vocal inflection as well has something to do with giving an acknowledgment that really ends a communication cycle. It is easy to demonstrate in person or on tape, harder to describe in the printed word. Generally, though, a downward inflection at the end of an acknowledgment is preferable to an upward one. The latter can be interpreted as a question and as an encouragement to continue talking.* Sometimes, of course, you will wish to offer such encouragement; we would simply advocate that such partial acknowledgments—a gentle "uh-huh?", or a quiet "yes?"—be used consciously and sparingly, and *never* when your client has in fact finished answering your question.

Overuse of partial acknowledgments is probably one of the most common mistakes made by poorly trained or inexperienced facilitators/therapists in running TIR, and there are at least two reasons why. For one thing, it is easy to fixate on the idea that the client needs to talk, to "get it out". But when we do that to the point of failing to note and acknowledge the fact that the viewer has *finished* answering our question or following our instruction, we lose track of the fact that it is possible, for all concerned, to have too much of a good thing. The pasta is *done,* and leaving it in the boiling water another five minutes will not make it better. On the contrary, if you permit your client's communication to simply run on—let alone to run on and on *and on,* unguided—you will at best be wasting his/her time and your own. If undirected introspection could have resolved the problem, (s)he would not have come to you for help in the first place. And in the worst-case scenario, by such ramblings (s)he will trigger other traumata or unresolved problems that you, still not having "tied a bow around" the presenting incident or theme that you set out to handle in the first place, will not be prepared to resolve.

There is another reason we may find ourselves substituting a partial acknowledgment for a full one: if we are not certain of what to do next, it is tempting to say simply "uh-huh?", thereby "buying time" by inviting our client to fill in the gap created by our ignorance and uncertainty, something that the client will almost inevitably and immediately *do.*

And what is wrong with that? Well, recall that we have posited here that the client, as far as (s)he is concerned, has in fact completed the communication to us. So consider the knot that we are *not* tying around the package. When we fail to give an acknowledgment that truly ends the cycle of communication for the client, (s)he will be prone to continue it; only now that cycle is no longer under control. (S)he is talking to fill a vacuum that we have inadvertently created, and because (s)he has already answered the question we *asked,* one (or both) of two things will happen:

1. (S)he will decide that we are not really very interested in him/her—if we were, we would have noticed that (s)he was finished;
2. (S)he will start to answer a question that we *didn't* ask.

---

* When you have found it difficult to get away from someone whom you find boring or overly garrulous, chances are that your acknowledgments have not been full acknowledgments, but rather ones that had a sort of bored, upward inflection at the end: "Uh-*huh?*" "*Yes?*" What you mean to do is to ask the person to get to the point, but such partial acknowledgments have exactly the opposite effect. They encourage the speaker to keep talking! A full acknowledgment, on the other hand, lets him/her know that (s)he has been heard. It creates closure.

And in allowing that to happen, again, we risk either his/her simply wasting his/her time and ours by talking about material that will help neither of us to resolve the case,* or his/her becoming caught up in an area of emotional charge that has little or nothing to do with the focus of the present session and one that we are not prepared to address at the moment. If we address the new focus, we would have to leave the actual agreed-upon target of the session—the presenting incident or theme—still triggered and unresolved.

Finally, note that the *tone* of an acknowledgment is very significant. If, for example, you deliver any of the acknowledgments given above in an inappropriate tone—such as with even the slightest unintended sarcasm or using false or inappropriate enthusiasm—it will just push your client's buttons instead of serving as a proper acknowledgment. The word "good", said in a calm, business-like tone, is often an excellent form of acknowledgment during a session; if said in a saccharin or overtly validating tone, however, "good" (or anything else, for that matter) is a very *poor* acknowledgment. Even a sympathetic tone can be distracting and inappropriate at times, taking your client's attention from what (s)he is viewing and drawing it to you.

---

* In the words of one viewer whose facilitator permitted him to continue without acknowledgment long after he had finished answering her question: "All that stuff I've just told you was just to tell you stuff. That wasn't new stuff to me."

HANDLING THE UNEXPECTED (Or, "What's That Coming Out of Left Field?!")

4

Different situation: female ... professional ... a secretary with management skills ... extremely capable individual, about forty years old ... husband an extremely successful doctor ... old home-town girl ... very efficient, friendly ... just a good professional, one that you'd want in the front office, someone who'd give you a good image with people coming through the front door. No problem whatsoever. She was operating in an office that had a management style that was based upon lies and mistrust. Employees were picked on to the point that this gal went from being that extremely efficient professional to being a woman who was afraid to type a letter for fear of making a mistake. She was completely dehumanized, if you will. Her sense of security went to zero. It affected her marriage. She was no longer capable of doing anything but going home and bawling by the hour. The agency where she worked had an Employee Assistance Program whereby you could call a number confidentially and you would get eight hours of professional counseling service. This gal sought that program and went through it. She was referred to a psychiatrist, and went to that psychiatrist for about four months. At that point, she came to me one day and said, "I understand that you have something that you have learned in California that might be able to help me ... and I need help." She was then still working in the same office, and had been threatened with probation—almost unheard of there.

When she came to me for help, she had also told me that her marriage was very shaky. I happened to know her husband, and the three of us agreed to meet. At that initial meeting, we set out the procedure. Her husband was completely trusting, allowing me and his wife to be in a room alone for maybe three hours, undisturbed, in their home. The end result of all of that was that two and a half months later, she went to her psychiatrist for her final session—her choice—and assisted the psychiatrist through the last, fifty-minute session. At the end of it, she said, "I don't think I need to pay you your fees to listen to your problems, Mrs. Psychiatrist, and at this point, our relationship is done, thank you very much!"

The lady subsequently decided to quit her job, took six weeks off, was hired back in another agency, doing the same type of work. She's held that job now for close to a year. The boss is extremely satisfied with her ... says, "Hey, this is the type of professional I've been looking for in my office for years and years and years!" One of her husband's comments sticks in my mind very clearly: "Thank you for giving me back my wife! Thank you for allowing her to have her life back!" A total success.

COMMUNICATION

This chapter is a continuation of Chapter 3, in that we will keep the communication theme. However, before we begin this part of communication, let us recall the basics of what you will be doing with your client in a session of TIR or Unblocking. In the main, you will be repeating numerous times a very rote question or series of questions and instructions, each time asking, in effect, that your client take a new and different look at the territory (s)he is exploring. It is important that the viewer be able to keep that up long enough to reach an end point, and yet (s)he may find that difficult, particularly if (s)he is new to the TIR procedure. You will be repeatedly directing the viewer's attention, after all, to areas of his/her life that are painful to confront, and from time to time it is likely that (s)he will cease being quite as cooperative as you might wish, particularly if the viewer is new to TIR. (S)he is likely to become "skittish".

Sometimes, too, when you are trying to get something done or get a question answered, your client (or whomever you are dealing with) will have something *(s)he* wants to get done or something on *his/her* mind which (s)he feels needs to be handled first or communicated first, before your cycle is completed. When such a thing is mentioned by the other person in the middle of your communication cycle, we call it an "origination". It is a *new* communication—a new cycle—started or "originated" by the other person.

If and when your clients originate during sessions (and they will), it is very easy to find yourself losing control of the focus and direction of the session, and it is vital that this *not* happen in TIR. This is because, as you will find, TIR and related procedures rely partly for their effectiveness on your ability as the facilitator to keep your viewer's attention tightly focused on a single, specific theme or incident—the target that both of you agreed on at the start of the session. It is only by maintaining such focus that you can be certain that any and all emotionally charged material that is triggered during the course of the session will in fact be resolved by the session's end point.

And how are you most likely to find your control of the session's focus slipping? Say, for instance, you are working on a heavily charged incident of childhood molestation of your client by an uncle of his, and the sixth time you ask him to return to the start of an incident, instead of simply saying, cooperatively, "OK, I'm there", he does something *else.*

What else? Practically *anything* else! And that's the point: what*ever* (s)he does or says will simply not answer the question you've asked, or represent compliance with the instruction you've just given. It will not fit the pattern the two of you have agreed to work with. You've asked your client to go to the start of the incident and instead of telling you (s)he has done so, (s)he says "No!" or (s)he tells you (s)he is about to throw up (rare, but it has happened) or he will say that (s)he "just can't *stand* it", or that (s)he has just remembered a special birthday, or even something that makes no sense to you whatsoever.

And when that happens—which it will, on occasion—the question becomes, "What do I do about *this?*" or "How do I get back on the rails from *here?*"

It is important that you ask yourself some such question. If you do not, the chances are good that you will rapidly lose control of the session and its focus, and that the "boxes" your client has been "wrapping" will suddenly proliferate, unwrapped. Too many topics will get broached, too much business left unfinished, and your client will find it impossible to reach the end point (s)he was working toward with you. You will be like the little Dutch boy with too many holes in the dike to plug up with your finger.

Imagine again, for example, that you have told your viewer to "go through the incident to the end", and that (s)he has been quiet for a minute or two, apparently following your instruction to silently review the incident. But then, instead of saying, "OK, I'm done", or "I've finished", or something like that—something you were *expecting*—your viewer says something like:

"I don't feel like looking at this anymore. I'd like to work on some issues I have with my father". That remark does *not* suggest compliance with your last instruction; therefore, it comes as something you were *not* expecting. What are you going to do with it?

What are you going to do when your client throws you the *unexpected* in a TIR or unblocking session, something that falls outside of the "script" you will be using? Well, if you do not mind "unwrapped boxes" and a lot of unfinished business left bobbing in your wake, one possibility might look like this:

Facilitator:	Go through the incident to the end.
Viewer:	*(At first silent, apparently reviewing the incident in his mind.)* I don't feel like looking at this anymore. *(long pause)* I think I'd like to work on some issues I have with my father.
Facilitator:	Tell me about your father.
Viewer:	Well, actually, it's not so much my father as authorities in general. Maybe we could spend some time on that.
Facilitator:	What about authorities?
Viewer:	Well, my sister was heavily suppressed by authorities ... the nuns ... when she was in Catholic school.
Facilitator:	Really? How did that affect you?
Viewer:	Not good; horribly, in fact. Her pain really hurt *me* ... but I guess I always had trouble with Catholics.
Facilitator:	Why was that?
Viewer:	I just never ... *You* aren't Catholic, are you?
Facilitator:	No ... did something come up for you that made you ask that?

What has happened here? The therapist has lost all semblance of control of the session. A number of things have occurred, none of them good or productive, and all of them preventable with better handling of communication by the facilitator.

The very first thing that the facilitator did wrong was to fail to acknowledge and then to query the viewer's unexpected statement, "I don't feel like running this procedure anymore". Instead, the facilitator simply accepted the client's statement about not wanting to look at the molestation any more. The facilitator passed over it entirely, just as if (s)he knew what had prompted it, and proceeded to take up an entirely new and unrelated subject, the viewer's father. Then, despite already having left one charged topic unhandled—the molestation, the original agreed-upon target—the facilitator accepts more instructions from the viewer and compliantly switches focus yet again. (S)he takes up "authorities", and then, after the briefest of one-question forays, hares off after a fourth and a *fifth* item, the sister's pain and then the "trouble with Catholics" issue to which the client's attention, now wholly out of control, has wandered. And at no time during this curious and unfortunate exercise has the therapist in fact *acknowledged* a single thing the client has said. So what do we have here in the way of open boxes?

All of the boxes have been left open: the molestation (which was the agreed-upon target of the session), issues with the father, issues with authorities, issues involving the sister, and issues involving Catholics! Any or all of those have the potential to be heavily emotionally charged. The therapist's permitting the viewer to simply dive in and talk about each in turn allowed each subject to act as a trigger for the next in line, and not one of them will be resolved in this session (or at all) if the therapist allows matters to continue as we have described them.

Take a look for a moment at the earlier parts of communications that we have discussed and recall what we have observed before about the "nesting" of the various components. Notice that more than one of the previous parts had to have been absent in the repertoire of the therapist here in order for things to have gone so awry—acknowledgment, certainly, but interest even before that. When the client said, "I don't feel like looking at this any more", the therapist failed to find the comment sufficiently *interesting* to warrant exploration, and as noted, surely should have. Any such remark from a client is highly significant in the context of a TIR session. This is not because it *explains* anything to you. In fact, it does not. Statements such as, "I don't feel like looking at this anymore", "I don't think we're getting anywhere with this", or "I'm too tired to continue", are not actually data; they are expressions of wishes or desires, masquerading as data. They tell you that *something* is going on, but not in fact what that something *is,* and you need to find out more if you wish to remain in communication with your client.

That your client does not wish to continue is not nearly as important as *why* (s)he does not. There are a myriad of reasons why clients might find themselves wanting to stop. They might simply have been momentarily distracted by something; they may have earlier reached a proper end point with respect to the issue you've been addressing, one that you failed to observe and to acknowledge at the time. You may inadvertently have taken up and be working on an issue or item that really is *not* actually of interest or concern to them and they may need to go to the bathroom. Or they may have merely reached a particularly painful point in viewing a troubling incident that they want to resolve, and have made a statement requiring nothing more than an acknowledgment and possibly gentle encouragement on your part. It is incumbent upon you as the facilitator to find out what *is* actually going on in any given instance. Depending on what you discover, you may continue, or stop, but it would never be wise to stop a TIR session (or, as in the example above, change the entire focus of the session) simply and only on the strength of your client's having said that (s)he is uncomfortable and/or wishes to stop.

A facilitator who understood the importance of that rule provided one of the videotaped sessions we use in TIR training. The incident being run was a vicious assault on the client during which she had been beaten nearly senseless by her father with an axe handle. At one point during the taped session, the therapist instructs her to go to the start of the incident* for perhaps the third or fourth time, and the client says, tearfully, "Oh please, doctor, don't make me go through it again".

What might we be tempted to do in such a case? It is certainly possible that we would feel an urge to comply with the client's expressed wish, is it not? In most contexts, to do otherwise would seem to be cruel if not actually dangerous. Not necessarily so in TIR, where it is not at all uncommon to find a sometimes hellish darkness before the dawn.

In this particular instance, rather than succumb to the temptation to let the client off the hook immediately, the doctor correctly assumes that there might be more to learn if there is a simple partial acknowledgment. Following a *very* quiet "Uh-huh", in a gently questioning tone, the client *immediately* says, "OK, I'm there". After several more passes through the incident, a marvelous end point occurs, with the viewer having achieved major, life-changing insight and enormous relief. "I think this is the best I have ever felt", the client says, smiling broadly. That end point would never have been attained if the facilitator had interpreted the client's plea to be allowed to stop as *data* rather than as a simple indicator that something *might* need to be explored. In that case, as it turned out, the plea was nothing more than a manifestation of the (temporary) difficulty the client was having in reviewing a painful incident. More exploration beyond that single partial acknowledgment was not required and would, in fact, have been counterproductive if attempted, serving only to take the client's attention off what it needed to be on in order to resolve the issue they set out to address.

---

* Again, that instruction is a part of the TIR protocol, and quite rote.

During the very first moments of the "long pause" noted at the start of the dialogue we gave above, then, the facilitator *should* have given a good acknowledgment and then immediately went to work to find out what had happened with the client to cause the statement about her no longer wishing to look at the issue on which both had "contracted" to focus! We will return to this below.

What is happening when the viewer states or otherwise manifests a concern? Typically, you, the facilitator, have begun a cycle of communication, but instead of simply answering your question or following your instruction and thus allowing you to complete the cycle with an acknowledgment and initiate a new one, your client jumps in with a comment or concern* of his/her own that has little or nothing to do with the topic you were addressing. Ignoring such originations gets us in trouble, both in and out of session. If your child comes to you and says, "Guess what, Mom, I got an A on the math final!" and you respond by saying, "Are you ready for dinner?" your child will not be happy. Your child feels ignored, and has been. And that is just one of an infinite variety of ways that one can mishandle another's concern. If you ask your husband what time it is, you have begun a cycle of communication that normally would be completed by his answer to your question and your acknowledging the answer. But if, instead of answering you with, "It's 2:15", he says, "I just spoke with my sister Marta and her company lost the funding", the quality of communication between the two of you will *not* be facilitated if you respond by persisting with your question instead of by addressing his concern.

How, then, do we deal with that sort of situation effectively, avoiding both the Scylla born of crudely ignoring a concern (as above), and the Charybdis we create when—in attempting to manifest a proper level of therapeutic concern ourselves—we allow our client to take over complete control of the session (*"You* aren't Catholic, are you?")?

The apparent problem is that although many aspects of TIR, Unblocking, and related techniques are indeed rote or close to it—in part for ease of teaching, but largely because of the importance of keeping the client's interest and attention on his/her mental environment and not on us—this particular aspect of managing the communication that takes place between the facilitator and the client does not lend itself to a rote treatment. Rote treatment

---

* When an origination from a viewer is about something that is not very important to him/her, we call it a "comment"; if the communication is about something that *is* important to him/her, we call it a "concern". The two are handled similarly, as you will see, but you will need to be more respectful of the latter.

would be possible if every client who became unpredictable could be relied upon to do so by saying or doing the same thing: "I don't feel like looking at this anymore. Maybe I'd like to work on some issues I have with my father", for example. But of course that would be predictable, and of course it is not what happens. In the immortal words of Gilda Radner in her role as Rosanne Rosannadanna on "Saturday Night Live", "It's always *some*thing!" And furthermore, it's always something *different!*

But there *is* a pattern, or algorithm, consisting of four steps in an easily learned sequence which, when followed assiduously, will always provide a means of completing a cycle of communication once you as the facilitator have initiated (or "originated") it. And that *pattern is* rote. No matter what unexpected concern or origination* your client may throw at you on a tangent, the following steps accurately outline the specific actions you must take in order to be certain of regaining or maintaining control of the session and of enabling it to reach its proper end point:

1. *Understand* the concern or origination that your viewer has presented to you.
2. *Acknowledge* it.
3. *Resolve* it (if any resolution beyond simply understanding and acknowledging the origination is required).
4. *Return* the viewer to the question he/she was to answer or the cycle you were trying to complete when the origination occurred.

Before we put flesh on the bones of that simple, rote outline, consider briefly just a tiny sample of the infinite number of concerns or client originations to which this would apply during a session of TIR or Unblocking. After silent review of an incident involving, say, a robbery, you ask your client to tell you what happened and you get one of the following responses:

He asks you, "Does the fact that I hate my mother mean that I'm sick?"
She tells you her stomach hurts.
He tells you he'd like to learn how to cook a decent omelet sometime.

---

* Bear in mind that your client's concerns will not always be spoken originations. An expression of pain flitting across his/her face unexpectedly, a twitch, or even a quick smile if it seems out of place in a given context, are also communications from your client that tell you there is something happening that you may very well need to find out about if you wish to stay in good communication with him/her.

She starts crying, says she "can't do it anymore," and asks if she may lie
down.

He smiles and says he suddenly feels as though his feet were missing.

She begins blinking rapidly for no apparent reason.

He says, "You know, this is a lot like taking Xanax."

She says, "Oh my god, I forgot my purse in the car and it's not locked."

In how many of the above cases would it be reasonably safe to assume
that we actually, fully understand what is happening in the universe of our
viewer without some sort of further exploration? Only one, really—the very
last, despite appearances to the contrary.

In that instance indeed, regardless of what reminded our client of her
oversight, she has made it very clear to us that there's a problem she needs
to handle. It should also be clear to us that as long as it remains unhandled,
all the client's attention will be riveted on it, and there will be none left for
the material we have contracted to address in the session.

So in that last case we have, indeed, completed *step one:* we fully understand the situation. *Step two* will be completed by our acknowledging what
she has told us.

The action required to complete *step three* (resolving the problem) is
obvious: she needs to run out to her car and rescue the purse. And when she
comes back, *step four*—returning her to what we were doing—would consist
of our simply reorienting her to the robbery we were running and to whatever
question we asked or instruction we gave her just prior to her origination
about the purse.

In each of the other cases, however, it would be a potentially major
blunder to brush off the first and second steps of the pattern we have
described above and merely to assume, from what we have been presented
with, that we know what is going on with our client.*

---

* Described in terms of the four-step pattern, the error made by the facilitator whose client
said, "I don't feel like looking at this anymore; maybe I'd like to work on some issues I have
with my father", was jumping directly to step three, and completely ignoring the first two vital
steps: understanding and acknowledgment. This is possibly *the* most common mistake made
by inadequately trained therapists attempting to use TIR. Made frequently, it will significantly
reduce the percentage of clients that you would otherwise be able to help with TIR. Too often,
in attempting to resolve something, we don't first take the time to be certain we *understand*.
We resolve something other than what we should have, and in consequence our clients, either
overtly or covertly, will begin to become uncomfortable with us. To however slight a degree,
we will have made the space unsafe for them.

What do we know about the client who suddenly wants us to tell him if he is "sick" because he hates his mother? Certainly not enough to know what action we should take next! The only thing we know with complete certainty is that we are *not* going to answer his question.*

Do we then simply ignore the question? Of course not. But we recognize it for what it is: not a question we should answer,** but an indication that something is happening that we need to get interested in and find out about. There are a number of ways we might go about this, including a "generic" approach consisting of the simple question, "What's happening?" When something unexpected occurs during a session, it is actually quite astonishing how often those two words from you will turn out to be an adequate and appropriate response, if not indeed the ideal one. In fact, that question might very well serve *verbatim* as our initial response to all but one of the six remaining concerns voiced or manifested by our hypothetical clients above.

The exception would be when the woman tells us that her stomach hurts. "What's happening?" would be something less than a graceful stab at step one. In cases where the viewer unexpectedly reports the existence of an unpleasant symptom, the first thing we need to determine would be when the symptom began. It could be that she was in discomfort before the session started—that she entered our office with a stomachache and that we have been attempting to run the session with a previously unrecognized (by us) distraction in place that will prevent our effective use of TIR. If so, resolving the problem (step three) will probably consist, at a minimum, of suspending the session until whatever the client needs to do in order to rid herself of the distraction has been done (e.g., a visit to her doctor, taking medication). It is also possible, however, that the discomfort is a physical manifestation of something that went on at the time of the robbery that she has been viewing—in other words, a symptom triggered by her review of the incident. If that is true, then the pain will have begun during our session, in which case it would *not* be good policy to stop the TIR. On the contrary, step three

---

* Why? Because to do so would be to interpret a datum and evaluate it for the client—actions expressly forbidden by the person-centered viewpoint and the Rules of Facilitation (discussed later) from and under which we must operate if we wish to be consistently effective when using TIR, Unblocking, and any other related metapsychological tools.

** Our failure to answer this question will not offend our client, because before we began TIR, we would have made sure that he understood and agreed with the rules under which we'd be working. At worst in such a case, we'd need to remind him of the rule as part of step three; in practice, though, you will seldom find such reminders to be required.

in that case would consist of giving the client sufficient encouragement to enable her to continue with the session despite the discomfort. What might that look like?

Facilitator:	Tell me what happened.
Viewer:	My stomach hurts. I don't think I want to do this any more.
Facilitator:	All right. When did the pain start? *[step one initiated: understand]*
Viewer:	I guess ... about five or ten minutes ago. *[step one completed]**
Facilitator:	OK. *[step two completed: acknowledge]* Remember we talked about how that kind of thing can sometimes happen just as a result of what we're doing in the session? *[step three initiated: resolve]*
Viewer:	Oh, yeah, you mean you think it'll go away of its own accord if we go on? Really? It's pretty uncomfortable.
Facilitator:	OK. Well, would it be all right with you to give it a shot even so?
Viewer:	I guess so.
Facilitator:	All right. Let me know any changes you notice as we go on, OK?
Viewer:	OK. *[step three completed]*
Facilitator:	Good. Remember where we were? *[step four initiated: return]*
Viewer:	Let's see ... I think you'd just asked me what happened the last time I went through the robbery.
Facilitator:	Right. Remember what you looked at there?
Viewer:	Yes.
Facilitator:	Good. Tell me what happened. *[step four completed]*

Typically, with the session once more under way, an end point will be reached by which time the pain will have vanished along with the rest of the symptoms connected with the robbery that was being addressed.

How might we apply the same four steps to the man with the omelet problem? Again, we need to take his statement at something other than its

---

* Having determined that the pain began during the session, we understand (step two) that in all likelihood it was caused by the material being viewed and will be resolved by continuing.

face value.* Unlikely as it may seem at first blush, this is another of the myriad cases in which, as noted above, we could easily get away with the simple question, "What's happening?"** Or we might say something a bit more case-specific, like, "OK, was there something we were looking at that brought that to mind?" Either way, he might mention some aspect of the incident he had been reviewing, but in any case the client would be likely to present us with sufficient data to understand (step one) and to acknowledge (step two) the sudden unexpected interest in omelets. In such a case, we could probably permit step two (acknowledgment) to perform double duty as step three (resolution) as well, and go directly to step four (return), with some such question as the one we used above. Thus:

> Facilitator: Do you recall where we were?
> Viewer: Oh, yeah, you were asking me to tell you what happened.
> Facilitator: Oh, right. Thanks. Tell me what happened.

... and we are back on track.

Regarding the melding of steps two and three referred to above, a separate and distinct handling (step three) is required in any instance where, having understood what is going on with our viewer, we realize that *more* needs to be done or said before the session can safely be resumed: the client needs to go to the bathroom, or to be reassured that we have duly noted a concern the client has raised and that we will not forget to address it in a subsequent session, or we need to turn on the A/C. Something beyond a simple acknowledgment of the client's origination needs to be resolved, in short. But often, as in the case we have hypothesized above, that is not true, and the only resolution (step three) required is a clear and unambiguous acknowledgment (step two) of the viewer's origination.

What about the next one—the woman who starts crying and tells us she can't do it anymore? Once again, it would be unwise in a TIR session to take

---

* If we *do* take it at face value, we will shortly find ourselves in the midst of a discussion about omelets ... or cooking ... or perhaps losses he has experienced as a cook. In short, we will have allowed the focus of the session to shift and broaden, willy-nilly, and we will no longer be able to contain the potential triggering within the boundaries of the single issue, theme, item, or incident that we have contracted to resolve.

** Bear in mind that we will carefully have gone over the "rules of the road" with the viewer before starting TIR, and that he will understand the importance of staying focused during the procedure. He will not *expect* a digression into the subject of omelets; if he is an experienced viewer, in fact, he will be consciously, as well as unconsciously, uncomfortable if you permit any such digression. Recall our earlier remarks about seatbelts.

this at face value and to simply stop the session. If we were not sure what to do about this, we could certainly get away with, "What's happening?" as our opening gambit. We might also say something like, "All right. When did you first notice that feeling?" The answer will tell us the most important thing we need to know, but with the question, we are also letting the client know that her concern concerns us as well. The viewer says, "Oh, about 20 minutes ago." Then we might say something like, "All right. Well, let me know about any change at all in that feeling as we continue here, OK?" We want her to be reassured and to know that we are not ignoring her concern. Chances are she will be willing to proceed at that point, and so we will go to step four, making the transition back to the procedure we have been running.

Do we know what is happening with the man who feels as if his feet are missing? No. We know only what he *says* he is feeling. We do not know what that means—whether he considers it to be good or bad—nor what caused him to feel that way. Do we need to find out? Yes! Could we simply ask, "What's happening?" Yes. It could be that he is experiencing a sudden and unpleasant numbness in his feet, something triggered by the work he has been doing or caused by the position he has been sitting in. But it could also be his way of expressing something positive, and hence possibly indicative of an end point's having been reached. It could be *anything* ... and we need to find out what, in order to know what to do next. So we might initiate step two (understand) with something like: "Hmm... could you tell me a little more about that?"

The same is true of the woman who suddenly begins blinking rapidly, and of the man who volunteers that "this is a lot like taking Xanax." Is the former fighting tears of grief or of joy or does she merely have something in her eye? Is the latter feeling numb and apathetic? or does he associate Xanax with peacefulness? We need to know. In the former case, "What's happening?"—or perhaps better (because less evaluative), "Has anything happened?"—would be an acceptable means of launching step two. In the latter case, "Tell me more about that," would be fine as an alternative to, "What's happening?"

SUMMATION OF HANDLING VIEWER CONCERNS

First, make sure that you *understand* what the viewer is telling you when (s)he says or does ("originates") something that departs from the pattern of the TIR or Unblocking you are using. Sometimes the meaning will be clear and the proper response obvious; often, however, it will not be, and you will need to explore, briefly or at length, in order to complete the step of fully understanding.

Second, when you have understood it, *acknowledge* the origination.

Third, *resolve* the concern or handle the origination. Do whatever is necessary to alleviate the viewer's concern so that (s)he can once more put his/her attention on your question or instruction.* This might involve completely handling the situation the viewer is concerned about, which in turn might include ending the session so that the client could see a doctor—which action would be simply a part of an extended step three. Conversely, a sufficient resolution might be simply to let him/her know that you have heard and noted the concern (s)he has raised, that it will not be neglected, and that you will address it when you have completed the item you are working on, or in a later session if (s)he wishes.

Fourth, *return* your client to the point from which you departed the procedure you were working with, and take it to a valid end point.

Sometimes the only thing needed to resolve your viewer's origination or concern is a simple acknowledgment from you, in which case you combine steps two and three and proceed directly to step four.

The need for correctly handling concerns exists in any kind of session and throughout all of life, but it is especially acute in a situation where, as in TIR, you need an efficient means of maintaining a particular focus in order to help someone effectively. If you take up every origination at length, you will find yourself chasing rabbits ("You aren't Catholic, are you?") and accomplishing nothing for the viewer. We have all experienced pointless and wandering conversations in which no single topic is ever covered nor any question resolved before another is introduced. Yet you cannot just ignore such invitations to detour, either, or the viewer will get upset. The solution is steps one through four: understand, acknowledge, resolve, and return.

And again, when you are not sure what to do with a verbal or nonverbal origination, you almost always have the recourse of asking the viewer, "What's happening?" More often than you might imagine, this is the best possible response to a viewer's unexpected comment, even if the comment takes the form of a question. You are certainly not obliged to answer any and all questions your viewer may ask (and often you should not). You can stay out

---

* Assuming, of course, that you have not found that the end point was actually reached earlier in the session, or that the issue you were addressing should not have been your target in the first place, and that it is still appropriate for him/her to return his/her attention to where it was prior to the origination.

of trouble only by *not* doing so. Even when "What's happening?" is not the most elegant response you might make, it will usually do quite nicely. At the very least, it is almost always a better way of buying time than is remaining silent or giving your client a partial acknowledgment.

Sometimes what a person expresses may be important, but it is not a negative concern. He may have something very positive to say about how things are going. For instance, if he says, "I just got the car back and damned if the insurance didn't cover the entire bill!" you would do well not to ignore this origination, or just to say, "OK". You would naturally want to say, "I'm glad to hear it!" or something of the sort.

In other words, if you wish to remain "real" to your viewer and in good communication with him, acknowledge his victories as well as the matters that trouble him. There is no rote procedure to all of this. The skill of handling originations is the skill of handling the infinite array of different concerns and comments that may arise. But you always have to go through steps one through four, above.

The key to handling client concerns and originations successfully is gracious parsimony. Ideally, you will do only what is necessary to smoothly return him to answering the question and no more; on the other hand, you must not be so brusque or abrupt in your handling that your client gets the idea that you don't really understand or share his concerns.

Cultivate the ability to handle originations, and you will tend to avoid being caught off guard or having your own buttons pushed when confronted by unexpected comments, questions, and expressions of concern from clients. In addition, your communication cycles will go much more smoothly. This skill, of course, is broadly applicable in life as well as in session. Couples can, for instance, derive enormous benefits from doing these exercises with each other under the guidance of one trained in their use.

THE RULES OF FACILITATION

5

An interesting thing occurred as a result of that. That lady was one of, oh, five or six that I had worked with at that point, all of whom, unbeknownst to me, had been clients of the same psychiatrist. All of them, also unbeknownst to me, had quit going to that psychiatrist after doing TIR with me. At that point, the psychiatrist came to me and asked what I was doing that was causing her clients to get well, and that whatever it was, she needed it. Well, the bottom line of that story was that I went to her and the senior psychiatrist in her office and we talked for a little bit over an hour. The gist of the conversation was, "We will be glad to bring you in under our insurance umbrella; you may operate with us." Their real interest, however, was, "How many clients can you bring into the business? Because we are in the process of building our client base...." It became obvious to me that their effort and thrust was not towards making people better. It was an effort to hook those people, to make 'em dependent upon that psychiatric business. Repeat business ... repeat ... repeat ... repeat. I decided that I wasn't "into" that kind of situation.

In addition to the markedly careful management of communication discussed in the previous chapters, the creation of an environment safe and nondistracting enough in which to do this work requires that the facilitator adhere strictly to certain policies or rules. Although some of them may seem obvious or simplistic* particularly to trained therapists, others are not, and their significance cannot be overstressed. Every one of them is

---

* The third one, for example, regarding confidentiality.

important and can be essential to the attainment of consistently successful results with facilitation.

Years of experience have taught us that the vast majority of all failures with TIR (and with the use of other techniques that rely on a client's attention being tightly focused) can be traced directly to violations, often "trivial", of one or more of the Rules of Facilitation. In training, we regard these rules as a strict code that one must abide by in order to be consistently successful in using TIR and related techniques. Dr. Coughlin (unpublished manuscript, Menlo Park, CA) stated the following:

> Initially it seemed impossible to me that virtually any traumatic incident could be handled using the same cues and without customizing the process to fit the problem. But customization, it begins to seem, is simply another way to influence outcome. Using neutral language to guide the viewer through the steps of TIR process facilitates the unfolding of a personal understanding. This creates the imperative to "stick to the script" in learning to do TIR. If one keeps to the language defined by the process, the viewer becomes accustomed to that language and is unlikely to attend to it. There is no distracting evaluation or judgment. Avoiding evaluation and judgment leaves the viewer free to follow his or her own network of associations. It frees the viewer to verbalize any material without concern for censure or approval from the facilitator.
>
> It must be added that it can also be very unsettling to viewers accustomed to more traditional therapies. I have found it necessary to stress the nonevaluative role of the facilitator in preparing clients for TIR. Still, some have pushed for critical commentary at the end of a session and were appeased only by the reassurance that I would comment at a later time if they wished. Rarely has a viewer ever actually requested such a review of me after the fact, since the process typically evolves to its own closure. More frequently, viewers will return stating things are better and that they are no longer interested in the material from the previous session.

There are 13 Rules of Facilitation, as follows:

1. *Do not interpret.* Resist any and all temptations to suggest what your viewer is seeing, or what it means, or may represent. Interpretation is the viewer's job, not yours, and it is vitally important that you regard and address your viewer as the only valid authority on matters concerning his or her own experience. It is possible and important

to simply accept and acknowledge the viewer's data. Do so! You are not required to agree with what your client tells you. Regard it simply as a statement describing another's viewpoint or opinion, and acknowledge it as such. Remember that over the course of a session, that viewpoint or opinion—if neither disputed nor reinforced, but simply acknowledged by you as facilitator—is very likely to change.

2. *Do not evaluate.* Negative *or* positive feedback is evaluative, anything at all that suggests—or might be construed as suggesting—that something the viewer has said or done has been judged by the facilitator in any way. The fact that such a judgement might be favorable makes no difference. In the context of viewing, praise can create negative effects almost as bad in the long run as those created by condemnation. It draws attention, and if we validate a given response or observation from a client, we must validate all of them, or risk the client's perceiving the mere absence of validation as disapproval. Successfully avoiding evaluation can be a demanding task, as even a tiny gesture or the slightest of smiles at the wrong moment can capture the viewer's attention and thereby take the viewer "out of session". Hence, in part, the importance of the early communication exercises.

3. *Maintain complete confidentiality of session data.** Confidentiality today can be a very complicated issue. Previously the complications generalized over what was said and/or to whom it was said outside the therapy session. These days we must be concerned with documents sent via the fax machine and e-mail; and what may be spoken over unsecured telephones (digital and cellular). We need to make distinctions between confidentiality, privileged communication, and privacy [7]. It should be apparent to most that no real therapy can occur without confidentiality. Therefore, we must each make ethical decisions about how to protect our clients and the information gleaned in our sessions.

4. *Maintain control of the session at all times, but do not overwhelm the viewer.* We refer again to the analogy of a seatbelt that restricts our motion to a degree, but which we welcome because it enhances our safety. Similarly, a viewer quickly comes to value the provision of a

---

* Again, this and certain others among the Rules would not be necessary to state if TIR were designed to be used always and only by trained therapists who could be relied upon to have taken, for example, a course in professional ethics. On occasion, however, TIR has been and will be taught to peer counselors and others who have not had such training.

relatively fixed and predictable framework by which (s)he is enabled to discover his/her own answers and insights.*

5. *Be certain you understand what the viewer is saying.* Never suggest or imply that you understand something the viewer has told you when in fact you do not. People tend to *feel* misunderstood when they are, and they don't like the feeling. When asking for clarification, always assume responsibility for not having understood; never imply that your viewer has been at fault: "I'm sorry, I didn't quite follow that", or the like, not, "That's not quite clear to me", and certainly not, "You're being unclear".

6. *Be interested, not interesting.* In some ways, this might be the single most important of all the rules. Your interest, if genuine, will be felt clearly and valued highly by the viewer. In some cases, it may be that perception of the facilitator's interest is the main thing that makes it possible to confront material (s)he needs to view in order to attain his or her goals. The facilitator who is interest*ing* to the viewer will significantly impede progress at best; at worst, and more likely, (s)he will render TIR and related techniques incapable of producing excellent—or even any—results.

7. *Your primary intention must be to help the viewer.* You can have other interests as well, of course—doing research or making a living, for example—but in a TIR session, the intention to help the viewer must be your primary motivation. Intend to help!

8. *Make sure that the viewer is well fed and rested and not under the influence of any psychoactive drug.* If your viewer is under the influence of any psychoactive drug that might interfere with concentration or dampen affect, or is at all sleepy or hungry, and you cannot readily remedy the situation—as by having the viewer get something to eat—it is best not to attempt TIR. As a general rule, when the viewer is experiencing any physical phenomena at all that might either dull or attract attention (such as physical exhaustion or an unhealed wound or injury causing significant pain), TIR is contraindicated (see Chapter Ten). An obvious exception to this would be if the physical

---

* Various schools of psychotherapy can be broadly characterized by whether they are or are not client-centered and/or directive. In a Venn diagram, psychoanalysis, for example, would occupy the quadrant labeled "Non-directive/Non-client-centered"; Carl Rogers' work, of course, would be "Client-centered/Non-directive"; Ellis' Rational-Emotive Therapy would be "Non-client-centered/Directive". It is hard to come up with any approach that is both directive and client-centered other than TIR and other applications of metapsychology.

condition were one that the viewer wished to address with TIR—a chronic, recurring pain, for instance, with no known medical cause.

9. *Make sure that the session is being given in a suitable space and with appropriate time available.* Do whatever is necessary to create an environment that is comfortable and free of distractions. Someone working with a lawnmower just outside your office window, for example, could make a session impossible for some viewers. If there is a telephone, fax, or other potential source of interruption nearby, disable or otherwise handle it before starting the session. As TIR sessions can be long, it is important that the viewer have a comfortable chair. See to it that the session will not be interrupted by a secretary or other visitor. Neither you nor the viewer should be under time pressure that could force the session to end or be interrupted prematurely. Whatever its obvious merits may be as a point of convenience in scheduling sessions and billing for third-party payments, the conventional fifty minute hour is completely unworkable in running TIR. Time is not a boundary issue in viewing. On the contrary, the possibility of your having to say, "I'm sorry, our time is up for today," while the viewer is in the midst of a heavy incident, will vastly reduce the chances of his trusting you enough for you to be able to help him. Simply consider that in saying such a thing, we are telling the client that (s)he is not as important to us as either our time or our next client.*

10. *Act predictably.* See our earlier remarks concerning "radar" and where the viewer's attention needs to be. And again, you may find it necessary on occasion to keep your next client waiting because the current one is running longer than you had anticipated. As noted earlier, this will not be a problem so long as the viewer in your waiting room is confident that you would not cut him/her off if (s)he were the one who needed a longer-than-expected session.

11. *Never attempt a session with a client who is unwilling or protesting.* You are trying to reduce stress in your clients, and coercion increases stress. If the courts or an outraged or overly solicitous spouse has sent a client to you entirely or even somewhat against his or her will, you

---

* In the words of one of the veterans French worked with who had had prior and extensive experience in an institutional setting organized specifically to treat PTSD, "I learned soon enough that you can't really get into anything [in a typical therapy session] because you only have an hour. You're in the middle of stuff, and the therapist would say, 'Hey, man, stay with that thought. I'll see you next Monday.'"

will be required to "sell" your work him or her before you do it if you wish to have any hope of success at all with that client as a viewer. By the same token, never rush a viewer during a session (see our comments about acknowledgment in the earlier section on communication). Your viewer must have good and sufficient reasons of his or her own for being in session with you. Finally, never take up an incident or issue because you, and not the viewer, have decided that it should be addressed. Only if the viewer's own *interest* is reflected in what you run will you achieve the superb results which TIR, Unblocking, and other applications of metapsychology are capable of producing; if it is not, then you will not.

12. *All your actions in a viewing session should facilitate viewing.* Most aspects of this rule might actually be subsumed under that part of rule 6, which states, in essence, "Do not be interesting". In other words, virtually anything we might be inclined to do that would not facilitate viewing—chatting, commenting "empathetically", "sharing", or "being honest" about ourselves or our own emotions as the facilitator—would also come under the heading of "being interesting". Any and all of the above will direct the viewer's attention to us, thereby removing it from what it needs to be on in order for viewing and the TIR procedure to be effective.

13. *Take each viewing action in any session to a positive end point.* Once again, take every effort never to leave a viewer "triggered" or "locked into" any significant degree of restimulation. All but invariably, viewers will arrive at valid end points within a single session of TIR if they are permitted to, and sessions that are kept open ended within wide limits facilitate this. It is your responsibility and not the viewer's to end the session at an appropriate time. At first, you may have to operate on pure faith that what we are telling you is true. Your viewer will in fact come out of what*ever* emotional "pit" (s)he may fall into in the course of running a traumatic incident with TIR, if you simply and calmly continue the process that would seem to have put the client there in the first place. After you have run a few sessions and are used to seeing the light appear at the end of the tunnel, though, your experience will give you all the confidence you need to simply continue when your viewer is severely restimulated, and to enable the viewer to reach an end point.

TIR IN DETAIL

6

New subject: female ... about 37 years old ... a son 15 or 16 years old ... in a situation where every three or four months, the person that she was dearly in love with would physically beat the crap out of her. He was into verbal abuse on a repeating basis as well. Such incidents would culminate in his moving out, taking their personal possessions, changing the bank account, stripping the proceeds out.

This particular lady had left a job in New York, where she'd been being paid close to $30 an hour in the engineering arena, to come to Idaho, where she'd accepted employment at $8 an hour. Her husband had been in some sort of security or law enforcement work ever since he had left Vietnam. He prided himself on looking younger than he was—a definite physical freak, a "hard body"—did a lot of weight work, never missed, two ... three ... four hours a day in the gym, and enjoyed trying to intimidate others. When she [his wife] came to me, [she] told me she knew that I'd been doing a lot of work with vets, and that some of them, who also worked for the police, had told her that I had something that was "pretty good". They wouldn't describe what it was, but they highly recommended that she ask me about it. She did.

Our first session was about two and a half hours long, and towards the end of it, she looked at me and said, "Now I know why I married that person! He is my father ... he acts like my father ... he treats me like my father did ... he abuses me like my father always has ...", and she went into about a thirty minute diatribe, screaming, yelling, beating on her own body, flailing her fists on her legs—at the end of which, she slowly reached a state of calm, with tears dripping and nose running. And in the space of about fifteen minutes after that, she looked up, her eyes opened, she smiled, and said, "I'm well. Thank you!" [Tape pause.]

"Hmm! I'm sitting here, crying like a baby ... grinnin"! It was one of the most pure, quick sessions I've ever given and, as I recall, that was the third time through the first incident that she picked to look at. She went directly to it. She'd been seeing a psychiatrist at that time for four months, three times a week, 50 minutes an hour. [laugh.] Oh ... and before she'd left New York, she'd been under psychiatric care for eighteen months there in one stretch. She looked at me and she said, "My God! All of that money, and all of that time, and I never got through to the issues." She said, "I feel like a brand new person! I feel light ... I feel like I weigh twenty pounds!"

Well, that story resulted in the abusive husband calling her and being informed by the lady that she had filed for divorce, that the divorce was going through, that it was not her fault—the divorce—that she had not ruined his career, that he had chosen to do that all on his own, that she was not going to kowtow to him any more.

Shortly after that conversation, she came bouncing into my office, sat down at my desk, and proceeded to tell me, in a voice that was loud enough to be heard fifty feet away, that whatever it was I had, it worked, and God-damn, she was glad to be alive again!

She has accepted employment at another firm. She has tripled her salary over what she was making in Lewiston. She left on the 20th of February, and on arriving on her new job, she picked up the phone and again thanked me, made sure that I had her new address and that she had mine. She has already sent a letter to me here in Stuttgart. She reports that her life is together, her divorce in progress, and she is ... in ... charge!

ASSESSING

Successful use of TIR depends on a number of ancillary factors being in place. We have discussed two of these at length in Chapters 2, 3, and 4. Here, we expand upon a third, assessment, or what might be called target acquisition. Some viewing procedures can be executed without reference to any particular area of your client's life.* With TIR and Unblocking, however, you will be

---

* If a client simply arrives in a session upset, for example, there are lists of questions (including unblocking) that can be asked very productively, each prefaced simply with the words, "since our last session", or "recently". As well, broad subjects such as communication can be explored with an interested client to good effect.

addressing, or "running", specific areas of the client's world—issues, or "items", that exist in the client's mental and emotional universe that (s)he knows about and is actively interested in changing or eliminating.

An item is a person, issue, question, theme, entity or incident that is accessible to your client and that may contain emotional charge. Working with clients to find an issue, item, or incident in their lives to which you can productively apply a viewing procedure such as TIR or Unblocking is called "assessing". Assessing is a simple activity, but one that it is essential to do correctly if you are to maintain the tight focus essential to the application of both of these procedures.

The concept of the "Awareness Threshold" [14, p. 409] (see Figure 4) is a useful one. It is a boundary posited to exist between those thoughts and mental images that one can readily call to mind and those which have been repressed to a greater or lesser extent. The Awareness Threshold is a speculative description or representation of a line—a level or degree of awareness above which all mental material is emotionally *un*charged, by virtue either of having been adequately examined, understood, and integrated at the time it was experienced, or of having been previously viewed and discharged. A client would gain nothing by viewing or reviewing such material. One's recollection, for example, of having gone to the theatre to see an amusing comedy is unlikely to be negatively emotionally charged. Assuming that the experience did not involve either primary pain—such as the moviegoer's having been mugged on the way home—or *secondary traumatization* [12] as a result of having been triggered by some event during the course of the evening. The incident should not pose a "memory management" problem, and review of the incident would be unlikely to bring about any sort of significant cognitive shift. It can be comfortably remembered, thought about, talked about, or forgotten, without consequence (e.g., emotional charge). In short, containing no repressed or insufficiently examined material, it lies above the line representing the Awareness Threshold (see [A] in Figure 4).

Just below the Threshold lies a level of potential awareness, in which level or band are found incidents and issues that are emotionally charged to a greater or lesser degree (see [B] on the left in Figure 4). These remain *partially* obscured to that same degree, but are, nonetheless, still capable of being viewed and, indeed, of being emotionally disarmed and fully resolved if approached in a safe space with the proper procedure(s).

Finally, below the zone of potential awareness lies a band of unconscious material which is not accessible. Issues and incidents that lie in that band (see [C] on the left in Figure 4) are too repressed to be addressed at all,

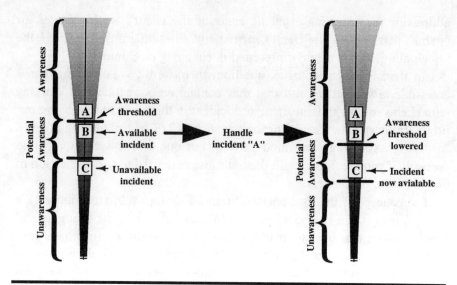

Figure 4   Awareness threshold, potential awareness, and unawareness. (Reprinted with permission from Ref. 13, p. 69.)

barring prior unburdening of material lying above it in the band of potential awareness.

Assessing, then, consists of locating areas in which a client has "memory management" difficulties—issues and incidents which cause the client pain or suffering, but which (s)he is willing to confront and is interested in viewing in order to resolve. All such areas lie, by definition, in the band of potential awareness. Below that band, the material is inaccessible; above it, there is no charge to be addressed, unburdened, or resolved. Thus, in assessing, we are looking for items concerning which the client will be found to know *some-thing*, but not everything. And given the client's interest, the facilitator's goal then becomes to address those items systematically, with procedures such as Unblocking and TIR, never permitting the session focus to stray from the one, single issue or item being addressed at any given time (recall our dis-cussion of boxes and ribbons) until an end point has been reached and that issue or incident has been resolved to the satisfaction of the client, at which point another can be taken up. Over time, of course, as items are addressed and resolved in session, the Awareness Threshold "descends",* and material that was previously unavailable can then become accessible for viewing.

---

* Or one might say that the issues below it—those that have been viewed and resolved—have "risen".

Assessment can also be defined as the action of finding "live" items, such an item being in turn defined as any charged issue or entity to which the client/viewer is capable of directing his attention. Typically, when that definition describes an item, the item will be one which the client will find to have an active interest in resolving.

Given the person-centered nature of the metapsychological approach represented by TIR, it will come as no surprise that the essential ingredient of any assessment is the viewer's interest. Therapists specializing in the treatment of posttraumatic stress will often find clients presenting with a fairly tightly circumscribed complaint, a specific incident—a sexual assault, for instance, or a robbery or traumatic loss. In such instances, assessment is generally a simple matter indeed. The client presents with symptoms stemming from an incident of which (s)he is consciously aware;* (s)he states explicitly that *that* incident is what (s)he wishes to resolve. In other words, there is viewer interest in it; so that is what you will address with TIR.** In other circumstances, assessment is more complex.

During an intake interview, numerous themes and incidents may be volunteered by the client, and assessment then becomes a matter of determining which item to focus on first. Again, the best indicator will always be your client's interest. If your client says, "Yes, *that's* what I want to work on now!" and none of the contraindications enumerated in Chapter 10 are present, the item you've selected will almost certainly go to resolution. A wrong choice, on the other hand, can result in poor or no results, because the viewer's interest will not have been captured, and the TIR procedure will not be taking you where you want to go. A case in point is that of Greg, a combat veteran, a self-described "troublemaker" during his tour in Vietnam and a soldier whose superiors had more than once assigned duties from whose attempted execution they had good reason to expect he would very likely not come back. During the 20 years subsequent to his return from Vietnam in 1968 at age 19, Greg manifested the full panoply of PTSD symptoms, eventually spending months in an inpatient program for treatment

---

* There are degrees of awareness, of course; we have found that the presence of debilitating emotional charge always depends on the existence of at least *some* degree of occlusion concerning aspects of the past event that gave rise to it, no matter how fully aware of the incident the survivor may *believe* him or herself to be ("I'll never forget the look he gave me before he...."). That occlusion is the target of the TIR procedure, and the fact of its lifting in the course of a session is manifest in the insights that are characteristic of a valid end point ("God, I'd completely forgotten that....", "*Now* I can see why....").

** Assuming, of course, that the client is an otherwise viable candidate for the procedure.

which left him—in his own estimation—no better off than he had been before he went in. During his intake interview for TIR, Greg listed a total of 51 discrete traumatic combat incidents, during one of which he had been wounded, in many of which he had lost friends, and in a few of which he and others had committed acts for which he had come to feel enormous guilt. The assessment in Greg's case consisted of simply handing him a list of the incidents he had mentioned during the initial interview and asking him which one most captured his attention—which one *he* thought ought first to be addressed. He chose one, and "ran it out" with TIR, reaching an end point containing enormous relief after a session lasting slightly longer than two hours. It was also productive over its course of a great deal of grief—grief no longer present, of course, at the end point.

At the start of his next session, his facilitator followed the same procedure, handing the list to Greg and asking him to choose the next target. Again, he chose "the worst one" (not previously resolved), and it was taken during the session to an excellent end point. In subsequent sessions, they did the same. This continued to be the pattern for some 12 sessions lasting a total of fewer than 25 hours. At the start of the 13th session, when his facilitator handed him the list, Greg looked at it for a long time, then expressed amazement and relief at the realization that although every one of the remaining 39 (as yet unaddressed) incidents had caused him grief and sleepless nights for years—indeed, he had wept while enumerating many of them during the lengthy intake interview during which he had generated the list—*none* of the incidents seemed any longer to interest him.* "I can't believe it, but that's really what it feels like looking at this", he told the facilitator. "Yes, it was bad shit, and it never should have happened. But it did...and it's over...and I don't have to keep living with it. I'm not the same person I was then, and it's not happening now. I'm *not* a bad guy...."

There is nothing particularly rote about assessment in TIR, but it is important to determine whether you are looking at an *incident* or a *theme;* as you will see, the two are not run in quite the same way. When you are working with a client who has suffered one or more major past traumata of which (s)he is aware, a unique event or events involving, for example, combat, rape, or torture, you will be running *an* incident, a single event in time about which the viewer can already remember a certain amount—perhaps a great

---

* Fortunately, that phenomenon seems to be common among survivors of multiple traumata; it is seldom if ever necessary to address every single traumatic incident in a lengthy, related series. Charge removed from those incidents most highly charged—typically the first ones run—appears to "bleed" the charge from parallel traumata, rendering them benign.

deal. How much (s)he is able to recall will vary greatly, but the point in Basic TIR is this: you will be addressing a *specific* traumatic incident that your viewer is aware of having experienced and that easily captures the attention. When such incidents exist, they should be addressed before anything else—given, of course, the interest and willingness of your client.

We use the term "Basic" to describe the particular variant of TIR that you will use to address such discrete incidents; "Basic", because barring complications, TIR used to address a single incident will be seen in its most spare and elegant form. Beyond those few rote questions and instructions necessary to bring your viewer to the start of the incident (s)he will be running, Basic TIR consists of just three instructions which you will be repeating sequentially:

1. "Go to the start of the incident and tell me when you have done so."
2. "Go through the incident, silently, to the end."
3. "Tell me what happened."

Basic TIR in practice, of course, can and usually does become at least a bit more complex than that, if only by virtue of occasionally demanding that the facilitator handle concerns originated by the viewer. Thematic TIR is inherently somewhat more complex than Basic TIR, demanding as it does that more than a single incident—each containing the same "theme"—undergo review by your client. A theme may be:

1. A feeling ("a feeling of uncertainty", "disappointment", or "the feeling that nothing matters")
2. An emotion ("fear of women", "deep apathy", "burning rage", or "terror of heights")
3. A sensation ("a tingling in the left ear", "disorientation", "a churning nausea", or "dizziness")
4. An attitude ("all men are evil", "you can't trust…", "they're all out to get me", or "inferiority")
5. A pain ("a sharp pain in the left elbow")

Note that these categories are not rigid. "Deep apathy", for example, might be described by some viewers as a *feeling* rather than as an *emotion*. In addressing themes, you accept whatever your viewer offers you, of course, without trying to sort out which category it "really" belongs in. The main point of having the categories is to give the viewer a point or area to focus on in deciding what he wants to change.

A word of caution: always use the exact wording that the client gives you in describing a theme. Don't vary it during your running of TIR or Unblocking, or you will not be taking advantage of the fact that those exact words can constitute a trigger leading to earlier material whereas other words, though similar, may not. If you alter the wording the client gives you, you may miss the chance of finding this material. "A feeling of not being able to stand men" may seem to us to be very much like "hatred of men", and the latter is certainly a bit easier for you as the facilitator to repeat, but to a client, they may represent very different states of mind, and both the theory of TIR and our own experience suggests that asking for incidents containing the latter will by no means necessarily enable the viewer to call to mind incidents that contain the former.

BASIC TIR

As noted above, although the patterns followed by the facilitator in both Basic and Thematic TIR are similar, they contain significant differences as well. For that reason, we present the two techniques separately, starting with the steps you will follow in running *Basic* TIR.* We have given each step in a shorthand form in **boldface** (as you may wish to abbreviate it in notes taken in session**), followed by an explanation. The viewing instructions you will give, and the questions you will ask the viewer verbatim are given in italics and in quotes.

INC

The first step is to find an incident to run. There is nothing particularly rote about this step. You will probably already have found the incident during the assessment phase. If not, you could simply ask, *"Is there any traumatic incident from your life that particularly stands out for you?"* (itself a form of assessment). Or, if the client is having difficulty in a certain area of his/her

---

* See also the summaries and flow charts for Basic and Thematic TIR.
** We would strongly advise that you do keep paper and pen in hand during sessions of both Unblocking and TIR. The kind and amount of notes you keep will depend on the needs you yourself perceive, of course, but at a minimum, you will need to write down the exact wording your viewer gives you for various items so that you do not forget them during the course of the session when you will need to repeat them more than once. As well, of course, you'll doubtless want to have the procedures written out and available to refer to during the session.

life—his/her work, for example—you could ask, *"Has there been any traumatic incident related to work that you are interested in looking at?"* Make sure you get a *specific* incident and not a series of incidents that has occupied months or years. The latter sort of "incident" (e.g., three years in a POW camp, or the major part of a childhood spent being molested) can and must be broken down into more discrete and manageable incidents. There is no hard and fast answer to the question of how long an incident can have lasted and still be manageable with TIR. As the facilitator, you are going to have to make judgment calls sometimes. To some degree, of course, it depends on how long ago the incident took place. A week-long incident that took place five or ten years (or more) in the past would be quite feasible to attempt in most cases; the same incident, if it happened a week or even a month ago, would almost certainly have to be broken down into smaller segments and addressed piecemeal. Otherwise, so much detail would be available and likely to be forthcoming that it might well take the viewer an hour or more merely to recount the incident once.*

There is one exception to this rule about not attempting to address a series of incidents all at the same time. This is when your client has a clear picture of the contents of a *type* of incident that occurred on more than one occasion, but is unable to distinguish one from the other because of their very close similarity, one to the next. In other words, essentially the same incident occurred repeatedly. In such cases, it is often possible to treat the events as if they had been in fact a single incident, and simply to run "that" incident.

Finally, be sure to check your client's interest in taking up an incident before you do so. You can ask something like, *"Are you interested in addressing the rape?"* or, *"Do you want to take up the time the sergeant on the wire begged you to kill him?"* If we look at running an incident as similar to playing a videotape, on this step you are making sure a particular tape—the right one—is loaded into the VCR.

---

* French discovered that fact to his embarrassment and sorrow very early on. He attempted to address as a single incident a traumatic divorce that had begun two years prior to the session in question and had yet to be finalized. At the end of an hour, the viewer was still going strong in her response to his *first* use of the instruction to "tell me what happened"! In that particular instance, the utter impossibility of what he was attempting was further assured by the fact that the viewer was still *in* the incident at the time of the session. A parallel example would be to attempt to use TIR in resolving the trauma of a mugging during the course of the mugging itself.

WHEN

"When did it happen?" Here, the answer that you want from the viewer is something that locates a particular event or incident important to the viewer—not necessarily for you. Thus, you don't care how loosely or precisely (s)he answers this question or by what means (s)he dates the incident. The viewer could, of course, answer, "January 8th, 1969", but (s)he could just as easily (and adequately) answer, "The summer I was in Canada", or, "When the guy moved out of the woods", or "Right after some party", or even just, "A long time ago". It seems important, though, if not indeed essential, to get *an* answer, however vague.

WHERE

"Where did it happen?" This question* seems helpful sometimes in establishing or refining the answer to the previous "When..." question, and like that one, it serves to put a subtle distance between the viewer and the traumatic event, thus possibly making the procedure feel "safer" to the client. Sometimes your viewer will already have answered the WHEN and/or the WHERE question while finding an incident to run. Instead of just having said, "Yes, [I've found an incident/theme to run]," he has said something like: "Yeah, I've got one...January 4th, 1969. That's when my platoon leader bought it." Or she has said, "Yes...Christmas day last year in my apartment". In the first of those instances, of course, you wouldn't bother to ask WHEN; in the second, you'd ask neither WHEN *nor* WHERE. (Though all the TIR steps were deliberately made quite rote, both for ease of teaching and memorization and because they work extremely well precisely as given, the intention was never that their use be robotic.)

LONG

"How long does it last?" Again, as in WHEN, you may get anything from a very precise answer to a very vague one. Take what you get, whether it is "47 minutes", "About an hour", or even, "Dunno, but it seemed like a hell of a long time." Do, however, bear in mind our earlier *caveat* about making sure that the duration is a manageable one. That point is one which you should clarify with your client before beginning TIR.

---

* Steven Bisbey added this question to the protocol.

START

"Go to the start of the incident and tell me when you have done so." What you want the viewer to do at this point is to "rewind the tape" to its starting point. But you *don't* want him to "push the play button" yet. When you are clearing this step in advance, make sure your client knows that you want him/her to find the *moment* that (s)he has decided the incident began.* You don't yet want the viewer to start looking at or moving through the entire incident. If you fail to get this point across, your viewer will often simply dive into the entire incident and begin to run it without waiting for your instruction to do so, and it is important for you not to let this happen. Why? Because one of the most significant gains the viewer will make early in the viewing with you is the growing ability to *control* the perception of the incident or incidents that have been tormenting him/her. In the past, (s)he has not been able to do that, but if *you* are careful to control the progress through the TIR steps, *(s)he* will begin to become able to do so.

AWARE

"Close your eyes. What are you aware of?" You use the AWARE step only when the viewer has gone to the start of any incident for the *first* time, or when the viewer has found an earlier starting point for a given incident and has gone to *that* for the first time.

In asking what (s)he is aware of, you want your viewer to perceive the "single frame" that is discernible at the *starting* point of the incident. The "pause button" has been pressed. You want the viewer to look at or perceive the scene, not yet as if it were a movie, containing action, but as if it were a freeze frame, however blurry. Most viewers will find it easier to do at least this step and the next with their eyes closed, and it is a good idea to suggest that they close them at this point if they have not done so already.** On this step, you do *not* want your viewer to report *action*—a "movie"—such as, "I see a man running towards me carrying something. At first I think it's the medic because I see something white on his head, but as he gets closer, I realize it's not, and that he's about to throw a grenade at me. I try to duck...to cover. I dive off the path, but....", or, "I'm aware of my father's partner coming

---

* Bisbey correctly notes that what you actually want here is the context at the start—the *normal* scene into which the first hint or element of the *abnormal* situation is about to be thrust.
** Some people aren't comfortable with their eyes closed, particularly when running something that is very painful, and it is OK if they keep them open. They may be able to close them later.

into the room. I get out of my bed and try to run into the bathroom...he gets between me and the door and...." Rather, as the viewer is telling you what (s)he is aware of, you want the concentration to be on nouns rather than verbs; you are after a description, usually brief, of a single "frame" or picture, such as, "I'm in the kitchen and I see a man next to the tree outside the window. He's wearing a red coat and holding something in his hand. The kitchen door is open..." or, "It's not very clear; I think there's a dog or some kind of animal sitting by a door or entrance to something ...," or even, "It's hard to get much of anything...pretty vague...just have an impression of darkness and a feeling of tension...."

This step of the TIR procedure gives you and the viewer an agreed-upon orientation point or anchor, one to which you can easily direct the viewer to return later.

If you do get an "action" answer, your viewer has effectively jumped two steps ahead in the procedure and is actually telling you what happened. Let it pass, but as a brief addendum the next time you ask the AWARE question, add something *softly* such as, "... *just there, right at the start of the incident*". If the miscue continues to happen, then sometime before your next session or the next TIR you run with that client, go over that step with him again and clarify what you want on that step—the "*still* perception". You can even have the viewer ask *you* the question several times. As (s)he does this, make up answers some of which are "stills" (correct) and some "action" (incorrect) and have the viewer tell you which is which.*

It is not essential that the viewer report what he perceives as if he were seeing or experiencing it in the present—"I *see*...", "There *is*...", rather than "I *saw*...", or "There *was*...." Such use of the present tense is a good indicator that the viewer is really contacting the incident and not just running it conceptually, however, and you will find it to be a very promising sign if and when (s)he does do this.

GO

"Go through the incident, silently, to the end." Now you have the viewer "push the play button and run the tape". Ideally (s)he watches and listens to the

---

* Educating your client, of course, requires that you evaluate for him, so when you are doing it, it is important, as stated earlier, to point out that difference between the "hat" you are wearing as an instructor and the strictly nonevaluative one you will be wearing as a facilitator once you have begun the formal session.

tape on his/her own, not yet reporting on it, but going through it silently in his/her own mind, without telling you about it. (S)he will usually contact and view the incident better if (s)he *simply* views it without having to talk about it at the same time. Some viewers, however, have difficulty doing this step silently if the incident is too traumatic. They appear to need the support that talking to the facilitator gives them. In such cases, let them tell you about it. Perhaps on later run-throughs they will be able to go through the incident without having to report to you about it at the same time. If the viewer does tell you about the incident, of course, you would omit TELL for that run-through, observing the policy that you should never ask your viewer a question that has already been answered, or instruct him/her to do something (s)he has already done. (Note that it is *not* a good idea to permit your client to indulge in endless analysis of any incident being run—a *caveat* we expand upon below.)

TELL

"Tell me what happened." For a number of reasons, this is the most important step for you as the facilitator.* With the viewer's answer, you will be receiving a lot of data, not only from the narrative, but also from how the viewer looks and sounds, his/her "indicators", as (s)he is telling you what happened. If you pay close attention to them, those data in turn will generally tell you exactly what you need to do (or not do) next.

Unless you educate them out of it, clients who have had extensive experience with analytically oriented therapy have a tendency to try to *analyze* the incident during this and the preceding step, instead of simply viewing and then describing it. You say, "Tell me what happened", and instead of saying something like, "I was lying in bed...I've got a big stuffed tiger that I use as a pillow...and I hear my uncle's footsteps coming down the hall...and I'm scared....", your client says something like, "Well, I can't help but feel that somehow or other it was my fault...that I encouraged him. I mean, my mother always used to tell me that I was..." Permitting a client to do that on a regular basis is a critical mistake, and if you make it, TIR will typically work poorly, if at all, with that client. What seems to happen in such cases is that the analysis acts as a sort of cushion between the client and the emotional force

---

* For your client, the previous step—silent review—is the most important. It is that step that is most often productive of the positive cognitive shifts that typically accompany end points; watch your client's indicators carefully during it.

in the incident. It is a substitute for actual viewing—and of course, the chances are that the client will have attempted to "analyze away" the pain and suffering innumerable times in the past. In any case—both in and out of therapy—and if it had ever worked, the client would not have presented in your office with the suffering in the first place.

The word "viewer" suggests quite clearly what your client needs in fact to be doing if you are to be able to witness the remarkable results which the TIR procedure, done correctly, is capable of producing. You do not want your client to try to "figure it out" or "explain it" or "make sense of it" *while* (s)he is running an incident; you do want the client to simply go through the incident as though (s)he were watching or acting in a movie. Occasionally you will encounter clients who appear not to be able to "see" or actually visualize past incidents as though they were movies. It is not vital that they be able to do so, although it is probably the simplest way to describe what you want them to do. But if they cannot, ask them to recall what they had for breakfast that morning, or to tell you something they saw on their way to your office. When answered, simply tell them that *whatever* mental action they performed in order to be able to answer *that* question is the same action you wish them to perform as necessary whenever running an incident or incidents with TIR.*

The movie/videotape analogy we have employed can be carried too far, of course. As Steven Bisbey has pointed out, you do *not* want your client to simply and only dissociate during viewing, to be or become merely a spectator. It is important that your client actually contact the traumata in—and the feelings he experienced during—the incidents being run. Should you encounter a client who seems to be keeping an incident "at arm's length" in such a fashion, you may need to take action to encourage this client to actually make contact with it. A way of doing that which is both effective and consistent with the second Rule of Facilitation (the rule that forbids evaluation) is to add the following sorts of instructions to the TIR "script" as many times as it takes to get your client to actually become "engaged" in the procedure:

"The next time I ask you to go through the incident, try to feel what you were feeling at the time."
"See if you can make out/recall any of the words spoken in the incident."

* See Harris & Linder [20] for a good review of perceptual sorting styles.

For "words spoken", you can substitute anything else that would have been present in the incident: sounds, colors, voices and voice tones, physical sensations, anything touched, and so forth. What you are doing, of course, is gently encouraging your client to take more than a superficial "look" at the painful event (s)he is describing. In other words, you are getting the viewer into the actual sensations and perceptions of the event.

More often than not in Basic TIR, you will simply go through the particular incident your client has chosen to run many times until it is discharged. After you have been through it at least five to ten times, however, you may begin to think about whether or not you should perhaps be looking for an earlier beginning or earlier incident that may be bleeding its charge into the one you've been addressing. It is during the TELL step that you will need to be most observant of the viewer to see whether or not charge is continuing to come off the incident. The general rule is that, so long as charge is coming off the incident, you keep to the same incident. Some indicators of reducing charge are:

> The viewer's recall or perception of the incident is changing in some way. *Change* is the most obvious signal that an incident is reducing.
> The viewer has better indicators and is becoming visibly more relieved.
> The viewer is manifesting an emotional discharge (such as crying or expressing anger).
> The viewer is recovering more memory of the incident; (s)he is becoming aware of new aspects of it.
> The viewer is becoming able, or more able, to perceive the incident.
> The viewer is becoming more aware of the reactions (s)he had and decisions (s)he made at the time of the incident and is reevaluating these.

If none of the above indicators is present and you have already been through the incident many times, it is time to look for an earlier starting point or—if there is no earlier starting point available—for an earlier incident.

Rarely, you may encounter a viewer who, though very interested in addressing some incident, will nonetheless find it impossible to talk to you about it and will tell you so. Let such a viewer know that (s)he doesn't have to tell you any more than (s)he wants to. Inform the viewer that in the TELL step, (s)he should simply relate whatever part(s) of the incident (s)he can—even if initially it is nothing more than the color of the sky at the time and the fact that the doorbell rang. You will find that if you *simply* and *only acknowledge* what is told to you on each pass through the incident, (s)he will begin to feel more at ease talking about it and will tender progressively more data on succeeding passes. Resist any and all temptation to "reflect back"...to elaborate or expand upon...to opine concerning...to "actively listen"...in short, to involve yourself as the facilitator in *any* discussion *whatsoever* with your client about what (s)he is telling you. Simply acknowledge the actions and communications, and eventually, the viewer will tell you everything (s)he needs to in order to resolve the incident and remove the charge contained therein.

Why is it significant and important to go through the incident a number of times, rather than just once? Because when a person is permitted to go through a painfully charged incident only once, one of two things will always and observably be the case. Either:

1. (S)he will not really "touch", or contact, the incident and its charge, or,
2. (S)he will become upset.

In the first case, the viewer will simply offer you a "prepackaged", "sanitized", *confrontable* version of the story, much as we—even if we knew we were quite ill—might answer "Fine!" in response to a friend or stranger's cheery "social" question, "How are you?" In the second case, the viewer will plunge into the charge in the incident just as (s)he has many times in the past. As an "in life" parallel to this phenomenon, consider the case of a man who is out for a social evening with friends for the first time since the unexpected death of his much-loved wife. He "keeps it together" pretty well right up to the moment when someone comes up to him and says, "I was so sorry to hear about your wife's death" (the trigger or "restimulator" that snaps the traumatic event into the present), at which point he suddenly begins to sob. In neither one of these circumstances will the viewer discover or resolve anything. In the first instance, *nothing* happens; in the second, he contacts the incident and becomes very disturbed. But by itself, that is simply something unpleasant that has happened to him many times before. In short, he will not have been helped in either case. The proof of *that* is that he is sitting in front of you now, needing help. There is actually one exception to this statement: over time, experienced viewers may reach a point at which they are able on occasion to reach an end point and to accomplish resolution following a single pass through an incident. Certainly, clients familiar with viewing tend to move more quickly than those first being introduced to the approach.* By the same token, the former require less and less of the facilitator/therapist's skills beyond the simple, rote delivery of the procedure itself, with good acknowledgments and adherence to the Rules.

In Basic TIR, then, when your viewer has finished his answer to TELL, you simply have him go back through the incident again, and again, and again, using START, GO, and TELL. If, after he has finished, he goes on to start ruminating or questioning the significance of what he has just told you,** simply give a good acknowledgment*** and return him to the start of the incident with:

START	*"Go to the start of the incident and tell me when you have done so."*
GO	*"Go through the incident, silently, to the end."*
TELL	*"Tell me what happened."*

Each time (s)he finishes telling you what happened, of course, you acknowledge the response clearly, but you must never succumb to the temptation to comment upon or interpret what has been told to you, or otherwise violate the Rules of Facilitation. All but invariably, enough passes through the incident will result in your viewer's attainment of a good end point, with the charge gone from the incident and his attention comfortably in the present.

Look for Changes. Change of *any* kind is what will tell you that you are on the right track in continuing to take a viewer repeatedly through a given narrative incident. It can be change in the *content* of the incident that she gives you in response to TELL—more or different characters appearing in

---

* The shortest TIR session that either of the present authors has ever given that resulted in full resolution of a significant trauma took slightly less than five minutes from start to finish. The viewer was working with French, and was a combat vet who had previously had some fifty hours of various viewing procedures, including a lot of TIR. His first session of TIR had taken well over two hours.

** Be careful to differentiate between idle rumination—speculation about the incident that seems to be going nowhere—and the sort of thinking out loud that often constitutes a part of an end point. The latter generally has a sort of *"Aha!"* feeling about it, or, *"I wonder if* that *might be the reason?!"*—something you would naturally associate with dawning insight—whereas the former sounds as though it is unlikely to lead to any happy conclusion. And indeed, as we noted earlier, it never does.

*** Recall the number of ways an acknowledgment can be *bad*. When a viewer starts to "ramble" unproductively, it is generally because the facilitator's acknowledgments are badly timed (too slow), or too soft, or inappropriately inflected—the facilitator's tone suggests that she wants to hear more, rather than that she has heard and wishes to acknowledge everything.

the incident, the scene being described from a different viewpoint, the viewer's perception that, "It seems as though maybe George was actually *behind* the door," "I'm actually not sure it *was* George that did it; maybe it was *Greg!*" or even, "God, I'm beginning to see how painful that actually was!" All such changes in the narrative content suggest that you continue running the same incident. On the other hand, the change you see may be not in the story content but in the viewer's *affect*—in the feelings and emotions that she manifests as she reviews the incident repeatedly. Thus, for example, though the narrative itself may remain relatively unchanged in successive passes, (s)he may begin by sounding and looking bored as the viewer describes the incident, then becomes angry during another pass, then overcome by grief in another, then rage, then boredom again, and so forth. And you treat change in affect exactly as you treat change in content—you simply continue to run the incident.

At the start of Basic TIR, it may require several passes through the incident, perhaps three or four, with little or no observable change occurring in either affect or content before the viewer begins to actually encounter the charge contained in it. *Then* you will see the changes begin during subsequent passes. Again, a sufficient number of passes with Basic TIR through a charged incident will almost always bring the viewer to a good end point. Keep in mind that the number of passes required will rarely be fewer than 5 or 6, will often be as many as 10 or 15 and, occasionally, will be as many as 20 or more.

On rare occasions, however, you may find that *after* having worked change into the running of a narrative incident, you *then* reach a point at which, although you do not have an end point, you have stopped seeing any change for several passes (at least two or three). If this happens, go to L/H.

L/H

"Is the incident getting lighter? Heavier?" It is possible, of course, to ask this as a single question by putting "or" between the words "lighter", and "heavier". The reason we have divided it is because it is easier to ask the question in that form without seeming—through inadvertently changing stress or emphasis—to favor one answer over the other. Asked as above, the question can be given without implication. All that is required is that we put exactly the same stress and inflection on each of the two words, something harder to do if the question is not divided. Most viewers intuitively grasp what is meant by this question; rarely does it seem to require any explanation. Even

so, make sure you clarify it before you start the session.* In essence, by "lighter" you mean: easier to confront, more interesting, producing better and better feelings, changing in a direction that the viewer feels good about. By "heavier", of course, you mean just the opposite: more difficult to confront, duller, producing more negative feelings, changing (if at all) in a direction that the viewer doesn't feel good about. Remember that in Basic TIR, you only ask "L/H?" after you have already gone through the incident a large number of times during which there *was* change. *After that*, when you get no change for two or three passes, it is appropriate to ask "L/H?" The fact that some of that earlier change will have been in a "bad" direction—towards grief, anger, hostility, etc.—did *not* mean that it was *then* time for you to do something new and different, such as asking "L/H?"

If your viewer answers "lighter", simply return to START, GO, TELL, checking the L/H question occasionally after any subsequent group of several passes with no observable change in affect or story content. In Basic TIR, if your viewer answers "heavier", you then go to ES incident.**

ES

"Does this incident actually have an earlier starting point?" An incident that does not resolve in Basic TIR despite numerous passes *may* simply need more iterations of START, GO, and TELL, but the fact that it hasn't resolved and is becoming "heavier" suggests that there may be charge connected with it of which the viewer is not yet aware. Often such charge, if present, will be located in an *earlier part* of the incident, a portion previously unidentified as such by the viewer, and that is why you ask this question. In addressing traumatic losses, for example, it is not particularly uncommon for clients to discover after a number of passes through the incident that they actually had a premonition of the loss before they witnessed or were notified of it, or that they actually found out about it earlier than they had initially recalled.

If your viewer answers "Yes", go to NS.

---

* In fact, unless you are very certain that your client will understand exactly what you mean by *any* word, question, or instruction you intend to use, it is very important that you go over them together before actually using them in session. A great deal of time can be wasted if you fail to do that—as by your client's taking the movie analogy too literally and thus deliberately running everything "at arm's length" in a dissociated fashion. (One inadequately prepared client, when asked "What are you aware of?" by her facilitator at the start of an incident, answered, "Well, I'm aware of the sound of your pen moving, and I can hear a car driving by outside." See Chapter 11.)

** Thematic incidents are handled differently, as you will see.

NS

"Go to the new start of the incident and tell me when you have done so." This question is simply a variation of START. You only use NS once, immediately after you have found an earlier starting point of the incident you are working on. From that point on, switch back to START. When your viewer has complied with NS, ask AWARE, then continue to cycle through GO, TELL, START, GO, TELL, etc., substituting START for NS from then on.

If the viewer answers "No" in response to ES, it is possible—even in the case of a heavily charged and apparently basic incident—that an incident earlier than the one you are running and similar to it in some way in the mind of your viewer has been triggered or restimulated by your running of the latter one. Granting this possibility, you go to EI.

EI

"Is there an earlier, similar incident?" If the client finds one, simply go back to WHEN (*"When did it happen?"*), and continue. Be aware that on occasion your viewer, particularly if new to the procedure, may initially be very uncertain about the existence of an earlier incident. What the viewer may get in response to this question is "just" a feeling, thought, or impression—or even something that (s)he thinks "must be imaginary". Encourage him/her not to invalidate such manifestations out of hand. You ask if there is an earlier incident and the viewer says there is the "impression" that there "might" have been, or tells you (s)he "can't really see one" but feels as if "there *should* be one", or even, "I see *some*thing, but I can't believe it's not imaginary." Ignore the uncertainty when that happens. Treat the answer as if it had been a confident "Yes" by simply acknowledging it and proceeding confidently yourself to, *"When did it happen?"* the next question in the protocol.

According to the theory of TIR, of course, the running of recent or more recent incidents in session has the effect of restimulating earlier incidents, if such indeed exist to be triggered. But incidents that are located far in the past, or have long been forgotten or suppressed, or which have previously been too heavily charged to be confronted, sometimes *will* appear at first to the viewer only as vague pictures, or foggy, indistinct impressions. It is easy—and too often a mistake—either to dismiss them on that account or to permit your viewer to do so, even if (s)he thinks it might be imaginary. More often than not, if you simply maintain a confident manner yourself when confronted by your viewer's uncertainty, (s)he will go ahead and look, however tentatively, at whatever comes up. And what starts out as a mere feeling or as something very unreal will frequently develop into a full-fledged and eminently "run-able" incident as the viewer continues to view it, not unlike a photograph in a developing tray in the darkroom.

When we discuss this point in lectures and workshops, someone almost inevitably brings up the question of false memories. We have yet to hear of an instance of false memories having been a problem with TIR, and suspect that there are a number of reasons for this. For one thing, while as above, we are prepared to ask viewers not to invalidate whatever image or ideation they "get", or that "comes up" in response to a question, we are not asking them to *validate* it either, and we make that clear at the outset. As the facilitator in the person-centered environment of a TIR session, you must eschew invalidation *and* validation, and simply acknowledge your client's communications. You want your clients to do the same—not to judge or to invalidate their own perceptions before inspection, but simply to look at, to *view*, whatever they get. Furthermore, because TIR is designed to be taken to an end point at which the issue addressed has been resolved, any "false" memory will have been sorted out *by the client* to his/her satisfaction by the end of the session, without any input at all from the facilitator.

Taking that matter a step further, what do you do if a vague and shadowy incident—or even one that she assures you that she can clearly recall—is labeled by your viewer as something that "couldn't have happened (or didn't happen) in *this* lifetime"? That question is yet another best answered by referring to the second Rule of Facilitation, "Thou shalt not evaluate". In other words, whatever your own philosophic, religious, or spiritual convictions, treat any such incident proffered by a viewer exactly as you would treat any other. Simply run it according to the protocol, and if something earlier comes up, run *that*...and all is likely to be well. "Past lives" may or may not be "real", or "valid", but if your clients regard you and your "space" as being sufficiently safe, and if you use TIR regularly, particularly Thematic TIR, you are very likely on occasion to encounter clients who will offer up such events.* Treat them differently than you would any other at your peril.

Sometimes the viewer will tell you that there is more than one earlier similar incident. If so, ask him/her to give you the one (s)he feels most

---

* Therapists and lay counselors with a transpersonal orientation have no trouble with this; some others do. TIR, however, only works up to its potential when the facilitator hews to the Rules of Facilitation. Those dictate, of course, that as facilitators—in the client-centered context that TIR and related techniques require—our opinions about such matters are utterly irrelevant. Whatever they are, they should remain quite unexpressed.

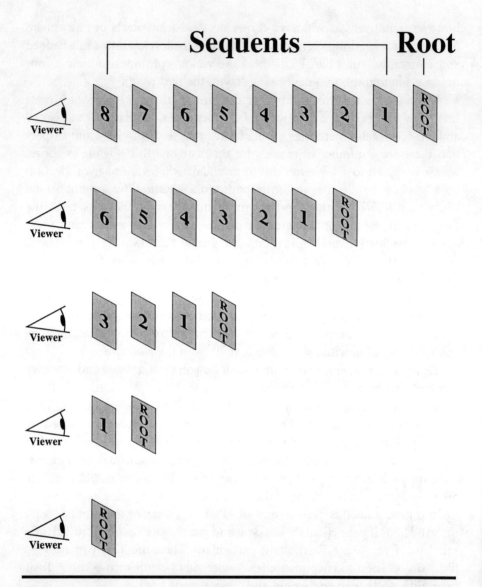

Figure 5   How to find a root incident. (Reprinted with permission from Ref. 13, p. 13.)

interested in or that seems most charged. If there is no particular preference, have the viewer give you the earliest one spotted—a rule that holds true for Thematic TIR as well.

If your viewer does not find an earlier similar incident, then return to START on the incident you have been running all along and continue as above. Bear in mind, though, the fact that as the viewer cycles through an incident, the charge is being removed. As (s)he does that, the viewer will either reach an end point *or* (s)he may find heavier and/or earlier charge revealed that was not available for inspection previously. And just because the viewer cannot find an earlier starting point or incident the first time you ask, doesn't mean that there are none. Perhaps, the next time you ask, or the *next after,* one will appear. Gerbode likens this phenomenon to that of a person attempting to view the slide at the bottom of a stack of color transparencies being held up to the light. In order to see the bottom-most transparency clearly, or at all, the ones covering it must first be removed, either *en masse* or piecemeal (see Figure 5).

When you competently manage communication in the session and adhere strictly to the Rules of Facilitation, the Basic TIR procedure described above will produce the desired result: a person whose thoughts, emotions, and behavior in the present are no longer adversely affected by the past traumas (s)he has experienced.

Basic TIR Steps—Summary (see Figure 6)

INC	Find an incident to run.
WHEN	*"When did it happen?"*
WHERE	*"Where did it happen?"*
LONG	*"How long does it last?"*
START	*"Go to the start of the incident and tell me when you have done so."*
AWARE	[if necessary, say: *"Close your eyes."*] then *"What are you aware of?"*
GO	*"Go through the incident, silently, to the end."*
TELL	*"Tell me what happened."*

When you have been told:

START	*"Go to the start of the incident and tell me when you have done so."*
GO	*"Go through the incident, silently, to the end."*
TELL	*"Tell me what happened."*

Repeat START, GO, and TELL many times; only then, if there is no change in either the viewer's recounting of the incident or in the affect:

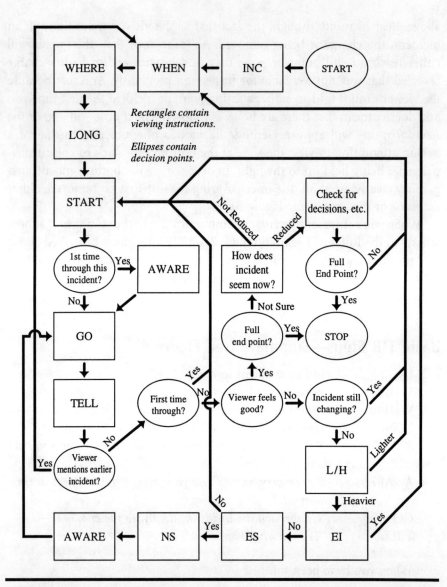

Figure 6   Thematic TIR flow chart. (Reprinted with permission from Ref. 13, p. 81.)

L/H   *"Is the incident getting lighter or heavier?"*

If "lighter", return to START; if "heavier", or "the same", or "I don't know":

ES   *"Does this incident actually have an earlier starting point?"*

If there is an earlier starting point, tell the viewer to:

NS   *"Go to the new start of the incident, and tell me when you have done so."*

and continue with AWARE, GO, and TELL when (s)he has done so. If there is no earlier starting point:

EI   *"Is there an earlier similar incident?"*

If there is an earlier incident, go to WHEN regarding that incident. If there is no earlier incident, then simply return to START on the incident you have been running.

THEMATIC TIR

A theme, as we stated earlier, is a feeling, emotion, sensation, attitude, or pain that a viewer is prone to having and doesn't want, and that has appeared in a *sequence* of two or more incidents ("sequents") in the viewer's past. The theme will be present in every incident in a sequence, although the theme itself is not the "glue" that holds them together, so to speak, or that created the sequence. That role is played by the charge in the original, "root" incident, and by the environmental triggers that restimulate that charge (see Figure 2 in Chapter 2). Restimulators are always similar from one sequent to the next, though they are not necessarily similar from beginning to end of the entire sequence. In a long sequence, in fact, it is unlikely that any given trigger will be found common to all of the sequents. Indeed, given our ability as human beings to associate and generalize, it is quite possible that later (more recent) incidents in a lengthy sequence will have *no* identifiable environmental triggers in common with the earliest one or ones. Again, referring to Figure 2 (in Chapter 2), elements contained in the original incident depicted* include a helicopter, children, an explosion (or loud noise), chewing gum (or its taste), and a tree line. Any one or more of those might, if encountered at a

---

* This was taken from an actual Vietnam combat incident run in a TIR session by French; none of the elements shown (with the exception of children) was uncommon in combat incidents in that country, especially lines of trees, often employed as ambush sites. Ask a combat vet from that war how he feels today about walking in the open near the edge of tree stands or forests.

later time and in a different place, act as a trigger for the rage that is the theme—the primary emotion experienced by the viewer at the time of the original incident, and the one present in every one of the sequents that sprang from that root. Moving further down the sequence, we see the triggers contained in the root incident becoming associated with other elements in later incidents—elements that were not present at all in the root incident, but which later come, themselves, to act as triggers. As noted earlier, by the time we reach the last incident depicted in the sequence, *none* of the triggers that restimulated it were elements present in the original, root, incident.

This fact has at least two important implications: for one thing, it explains why, for example, when asked by the facilitator to find an incident containing "a feeling of total worthlessness", the viewer will almost *never* go directly to the basic or "root" incident of the Thematic sequence, despite the fact that that would certainly be the most efficient way to address the theme. For another, it is the reason why it is sometimes virtually impossible for either the facilitator *or* the viewer to recognize—at least initially—the *similarity* between an incident just viewed and another that "just comes to mind" when the facilitator asks if there is an earlier, similar incident. This, in turn, is why it is so important that neither you as the facilitator nor your viewer invalidate any answer that may come up when you ask the ES question on such grounds as: "I can't see any similarity between what I got when you asked if there was an earlier starting point, and what I've just been going over." It may take several passes through such an earlier incident before its relevance becomes apparent. Typically, if you ask the question and your viewer immediately finds him/herself looking at "something that just came to mind", viewing rather than rejecting whatever the "something" is will turn out to be productive. The question, *"Is there an earlier, similar incident?"** itself seems to act as a trigger, and what*ever* it triggers is what should be looked at next.

The technique used in running Thematic TIR is quite similar to that of Basic TIR, but there are some significant differences, described below.

INC

Given the opportunity, you will generally wish to address specific traumatic incidents before taking up themes. This is because the former will tend to have, if not the heaviest charge, at least the most readily available. If a client presents with a theme, then, ask him/her if (s)he is aware of any specific

---

* Alternatively, in the case of Thematic TIR, *"Is there an earlier incident containing* [theme]*?"*

incident that originally gave rise to that theme. If the viewer comes to you with a fear of flying that is preventing him/her from being able to function effectively at work, for example, ask if (s)he is aware of any particular incident that might have caused the feeling. If you hear something like, "Oh, yes, I crashed in a plane five years ago and have had a terror of them ever since", you have an incident which (s)he will very likely be interested in running out with Basic TIR and one which, when run, will all but certainly eliminate the theme—the fear of flying.

But it may be that (s)he is aware of no such basic incident. In that case, you will simply run the theme as a theme, the first difference being that you will be asking not for a specific, known event—*the* incident—but, rather, for *an* incident containing the theme. Instruct your viewer, then, to *"Find an incident containing* [viewer's wording of the theme]*"*. Again, make sure you have a *specific* incident, not the viewer's whole life or a significant portion of it.

The words in brackets above are important. Whenever you ask for or otherwise refer to a theme or other item, it is important that you employ the exact wording used by your client in referring to it. This is because triggers can be very precise. "Hatred of men" may seem to me to be pretty much the same thing as "a feeling of not being able to stand men", and it is certainly easier to say, but the two wordings may convey very different messages to my client. If the latter is the wording your client used in volunteering the item in the first place, then you would be well advised to stick to it. The only apparent exception to this rule is found when a volunteered item is simply too unwieldy to insert in a viewing instruction that you will be repeating numerous times. Both you and your client would likely find the question, *"Is there an earlier incident containing the feeling that anytime I find myself having to deal with my father, or my boss, or a policeman, or anyone like that at all, that I'm going to just fall apart and lose it right there?"* rather too cumbersome to use repeatedly. Yet that may be the exact wording of the theme that you first got from your viewer. In such a case, do not decide unilaterally that a better wording would be "Fear of authority figures" and attempt to run that. Rather, ask your viewer if (s)he can summarize the theme in, say, five or ten words or less. (S)he might say, "Oh, sure. It boils down to 'Terror around authorities.'" Use *that* wording!

Once you've established the theme and the first incident you will run as above, the next several steps you will use are identical to the steps in Basic TIR: WHEN?, WHERE?, LONG?, START, AWARE?, GO, and TELL.

The major differences in running Thematic and Basic TIR first become apparent after the second TELL of the TIR procedure. In Basic TIR, you would virtually *never* ask for an earlier incident or use L/H (*"Is the incident getting lighter or heavier?"*) at this point. In Thematic TIR, you *often* do without first running through an incident many times. This is because, again, it is almost always very safe to assume that your client will not have started out by running the earliest incident (s)he actually experienced that contains the theme, particularly if (s)he is relatively inexperienced as a viewer. Often—as when a theme is one your client has had since childhood and the first incident (s)he selects took place a week ago—you will know for a fact that (s)he has not. In which case, you can skip asking "L/H" and go directly to EI. In any event, the chances are excellent that if the answer to L/H is "heavier", it will be because viewing the current incident has restimulated an earlier one, as yet unexamined. More often than not, (s)he will now be able to find this earlier incident if you ask him/her to look for it. So if the current incident is getting heavier, or you know for a fact that there must be one or more earlier incidents, you simply ask EI (*"Is there an earlier incident containing* [theme]*?"*). If (s)he finds an earlier incident, simply go to WHEN on this new incident and continue with WHERE?, LONG?, START, and so on. If (s)he cannot yet see or get any impression of an earlier incident containing the theme, you *then* go to ES (*"Does this incident actually have an earlier starting point?"*) and, if it does, continue with NS (*"Go to the new start of the incident."*), AWARE, GO, TELL, START, GO, TELL, etc.

Note that the sequence in which you ask EI and ES in Thematic TIR is the reverse of that given in Basic TIR, where first you asked for ES and only then—if there was no earlier start—for an EI. The reason for this is because in each case, in the interests of efficiency, you ask the question first that is most likely to be productive of a positive answer.

Thematic TIR Steps—Summary (see Figure 7)

First, establish a theme that the viewer wants to run. Then run it as follows:

INC	*"Find an incident containing* [theme, in viewer's words]*."*
WHEN	*"When did it happen?"*
WHERE	*"Where did it happen?"*
LONG	*"How long does it last?"*
START	*"Go to the start of the incident and tell me when you have done so."*

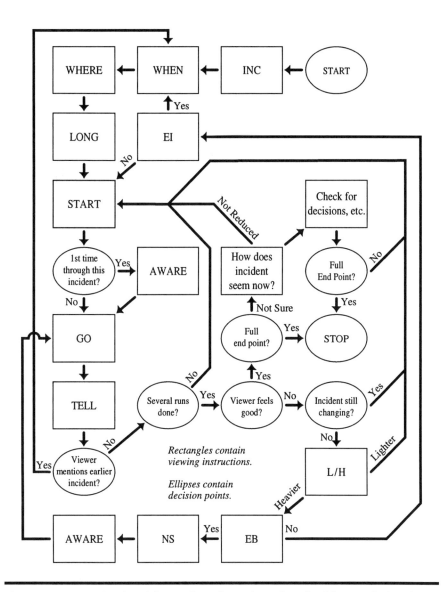

Figure 7   Narrative (Basic) TIR flowchart. (Reprinted with permission from Ref. 13, p. 80.)

AWARE	[if necessary, say: *"Close your eyes."*] then *"What are you aware of?"*
GO	*"Go through the incident, silently, to the end."*
TELL	*"Tell me what happened."*

When (s)he has told you:

START   *"Go to the start of the incident and tell me when you have done so."*
GO   *"Go through the incident, silently, to the end."*
TELL   *"Tell me what happened."*

If no significant change after the second or subsequent iterations, and the incident you are dealing with could conceivably be the root of the sequence:

L/H   *"Is the incident getting lighter or heavier?"*

If "lighter", return to START; if "heavier", or "the same", or "I don't know", or if you know there's an earlier incident:

EI   *"Is there an earlier incident containing* [theme, in viewer's words]*?"*

If there is an earlier incident, go to WHEN and continue with that incident. If not:

ES   *"Does this incident actually have an earlier starting point?"*

If there is an earlier starting point:

NS   *"Go to the new start of the incident and tell me when you have done so."*

and continue with AWARE, GO, TELL, etc.
If there is no earlier starting point, just return to START.

OPTIONAL ADDITIONAL TIR QUESTIONS

The TIR "script", run exactly as described earlier in this chapter, will generally produce excellent results and end points in a very large majority of viewers whom you have properly screened and prepared to run the procedure. On rare occasions, however, you may find yourself working with a viewer who appears to have bled all the charge from (or "flattened") an incident, but who nonetheless has not attained a full end point—this, despite the fact that you asked "How does the incident seem?" and inquired after conclusions (s)he reached or decisions (s)he might have made at the time of the incident. On occasion as well, particularly though not exclusively when your viewer is inexperienced in running TIR, you may find as suggested earlier that (s)he is running an incident at arm's length, as it were, and not contacting the actual pain or emotional impact it contains, but only its cognitive aspects. Again, such a client seems to regard the incident from a dissociated viewpoint, never really seeming to be personally involved in the event but reporting it exclusively as if (s)he were a mere observer. Rarely, too, you may encounter the reverse of this: a viewer who despite contacting the emotional content of an incident never makes any significant cognitive or emotional shift. For any of those cases, the additional questions listed below should be helpful. They should be regarded as adjunctive to and *not* as a regular part of the TIR procedure, but when used judiciously and selectively, and non-robotically—as appropriate to the particular *lacuna* you have noted in your viewer's running of the incident—you may find them valuable. You should not have to use any of these questions frequently or—ever—as substitutes for any of the standard questions or instructions given earlier.

[If the viewer has not told you] What were you doing during the incident?
What were you thinking at the time?
Did you form any conclusions at that time?
Did you believe there was a threat or potential threat to you at that time?
Was there anything you believed was going to happen at that time?
What were you feeling at that time?
Did you express it?
How? (This one and the previous two are three separate questions.)
How did you react at the time?
Was there anything you wanted to say at the time and didn't?
Was there anything you think you should have said at the time and didn't?
Were you unwilling to be, or remain, where you were at that time?
Did you have any impulses at the time—anything you felt like doing, but didn't?
[If not already asked] Did you make any decisions at the time of the incident?

THE DIRECTION
OF CAUSATION

7

Whew! I didn't realize that I had that much emotional attachment, in terms of pure, outright pleasure! For a male like me ... who went through the military ... who was raised in Montana on a rock farm, very poor ... who came up with somewhat of a macho image (if you were a man, you proved what you were, and you damned sure didn't cry!) [laugh]—it feels kinda good to sit here, and grin, and let tears run, and not feel bad about it.

Traumatic incidents contain action or impact proceeding from one person or group or source* to another—what might be termed "directed action". This admittedly somewhat awkward term connotes responsibility, or its primary location, but the two concepts are not interchangeable.

We have emotional charge connected, of course, not only to events in which we ourselves have suffered on account of things that have been done (or have simply happened) to us—things for which we were not in any way directly responsible—but there is also charge connected to incidents in which we:

- have been the perpetrator of harm to others
- have witnessed or otherwise come to know of others harming others
- have harmed ourselves

The four principal directions in which an action or causation can "flow", then, are:

---

* Nature or accident, of course, can be the cause of a trauma.

Inflow	Something happening to the viewer as the direct result of the action of someone or something else (e.g., the viewer was attacked by a mugger).
Outflow	The viewer causing something to happen to someone or something else (e.g., the viewer attacked and beat a classmate when he was in school).
Crossflow	The viewer observing (or otherwise affected by) something done to others by others (e.g., the viewer witnesses her mother being attacked and beaten by her father).
Reflexive flow	The viewer does something to him/herself (e.g., the viewer breaks his own hand by hitting a door with his fist in a rage).

Without question, inflow is the direction of causation that you will find yourself presented with most often by clients. Though many traumatized clients do present with outflow incidents (e.g., perpetrators), crossflow incidents (e.g., rescue workers, distraught parents), and reflexive flow incidents (e.g., self-inflicted injuries), a majority will present with incidents containing physical and/or emotional pain that has been inflicted on them by other people or external forces.

Whatever flow you are initially presented with and resolve, it can be a good idea subsequently to inquire after the remaining flows that you have not addressed, and to determine if any of them are charged in your viewer's estimation. On occasion, you will find that one or more of them will be, and when that is the case, it is important to run them.

When we consult the client's interest, flows seem to present themselves in the order in which it is necessary and possible to address them. Inflow incidents tend to be the first to appear, and it seems logical and intuitively correct that this should be the case. When we do something to another or others (outflow) that subsequently causes us—or would normally cause us—to experience feelings of guilt, we frequently do so on account of having undergone one or more real or apparent threats to our own survival or well-being. When unexamined, these threats seem to justify or motivate—if not indeed to mandate—our own harmful action(s).* When this is the case, we feel accused and defensive if asked for something harmful we may have done to another unless we have first been given the opportunity to address and

---

* Abusers, of course, have often been abused themselves.

fully resolve the charge contained in incidents of another or others doing things to us.*

For a possibly amusing but nonetheless valid instance of this phenomena, consider attempting to force a ten o'clock scholar to recognize the error of his ways. His parents and teachers tell him that he is wrong to be perennially late, that it's important not to miss class, that other kids manage to be on time, that his grades will suffer, and so forth. Perhaps they ask or demand that he tell them the reasons why it is a bad idea to be late, or attempt to force a promise that he will start arriving on time.

What are we doing? We're trying to get him to confront the second flow—his doing something wrong or hurtful**—before giving him a chance to look at his motivations (the inflow). In addition to making a very unsafe and accusatory space, all of our efforts miss the point, the student is being late to school because at some unexamined level he has decided that it is right to be late, and that there is adequate justification for it—some reason it is "OK" to be late. And if we wish to change his mind and hence his behavior, pointing out the error of his ways is not usually the best way to go about it.

A good way to do it is to ask him, sincerely and nonaccusatorily, to tell us, or to write a list, of all the reasons why it is in fact a good idea for him to be late. If he says, "Oh, c'mon, of course it isn't", then we need to respond with something along the lines of, "No, really. If it were flat out, completely, totally bad and wrong and there were no reasons for being late that made any sense to you, you'd be on time. We both know that. You're not stupid. So just humor me and answer the question. Maybe you haven't looked before, but I guarantee you there are at least some reasons why it makes sense for you to be late. I promise I'm not going to judge your answers in any way at all. In fact, if you want to just write down as many reasons as you can come up with and then throw the paper away without showing it to me, it's OK with me. But do it."

If we keep our word and simply acknowledge him for having done as we asked, we are very likely to see his tardiness stop. Given a safe space in which to look at—view—and evaluate his reasons for being late, he will (assuming they are weak!) tend to discard them himself. But if we succumb to the

---

* The present authors would predict with certainty that if TIR were to be used as part of any rehabilitation program dealing with offenders, it would prove essential to address and resolve inflow incidents before attempting to address the outflow events.

** Because ultimately he is hurting himself more than anyone else, it is also the fourth—or reflexive—flow.

temptation to bring our "wisdom" to bear on the situation and thus to evaluate or dispute the reasons he comes up with for being late, we should not be surprised if his response—overtly or covertly—is either to deny or to defend them.

Having taken an inflow theme or incident to an end point, then, it is sometimes wise—especially if the resolution achieved in addressing the primary incident seems in any way incomplete—to check with your viewer to see if there are any other charged flows, flows containing themes or incidents perceived by the viewer as similar in any way* to the one you have addressed. If there are, you would want to address them as soon as possible.

The woman who comes to you because of her suffering on having been divorced by her husband may herself have caused someone else to suffer in a similar fashion. The man who was bullied as a child may himself have bullied others. Unexpected relief can sometimes be attained by checking for such possibilities—always, of course, in an utterly nonaccusatory fashion.

In order to run TIR, you will have to construct instructions for the four flows. Usually but by no means always, as we noted above, the incident that your client comes up with first will be an inflow incident. When more than one flow is addressed, they are normally presented in the order in which we have presented them above: inflow, outflow, crossflow, and reflexive flow. But if your client's attention is focused initially on, say, an outflow incident—a distraught parent, ridden with guilt as a result of having badly injuring his child by accident, for example—you would take up that flow first, only then checking to see if there exists a similar inflow incident, then a crossflow, and finally a reflexive flow. If you happen to begin with a crossflow, you would next look for an inflow, then outflow, then reflexive flow, and so forth.

Crossflow incidents, of course, can be doubly charged on account of the loss that is often connected with them. Witnessing the violent death of a stranger can be highly traumatic; if the victim is a loved one, it is worse.

Interestingly, the fourth or reflexive flow seems generally to be the most difficult for us to perceive, possibly because it is easy to confuse responsibility with blame. On the other hand, some of the most dramatic end points and cognitive and behavioral shifts you will observe in using TIR will stem from

---

* Recall our earlier discussion of "similarity". It is important that the viewer understands that in asking about a "similar" incident, you are asking a very broad question. As a general rule—and always, of course, assuming your client's interest—you would take up *any* incident that occurred to him/her upon your asking the question. Often, the similarity between incidents seems to be perceived initially at an unconscious level, becoming clear perhaps only after several (or many) reviews of the incident.

your viewer's recognizing and resolving things that (s)he has done to—or contributed in some way to having brought on—him/herself. It is often the case, as well, that both themes and incidents that initially present as one of the other three flows—especially the first—resolve in end points characterized by precisely such a recognition on the part of the viewer.

This too seems eminently logical. Probably the most common intention found in painful incidents is the intention that "this must never happen again". But consider: by definition, we feel safe and empowered only to the degree that we are able to perceive ourselves as capable of influencing the events we experience. Put another way, as long as your client can see only the inflow in his/her life, (s)he will be unable to perceive him/herself as anything other than the passive target of always potentially harmful if not actively hostile forces (s)he does not control.

End points characterized by a perception of one's own responsibility (as opposed to blame) seem particularly empowering. Witness or experience one and you will see the transformation from victim to survivor occur before your eyes; and not merely to survivor, but to one no longer susceptible to restimulation by chronic triggers.

In saying this, we do not wish to suggest that the responsibility assumed by a victim for his/her victimization in any way reduces the responsibility of the perpetrator for the act. Again, responsibility as we are using the term is not blame. The latter can be assigned—and is, of course, in courts of law and elsewhere; the former cannot be assigned, only assumed.

Both Basic and Thematic TIR instructions can be put into four flows, and you are wise to address any flow that seems live and has the viewer's interest. Do not force other flows on the viewer, however. Only check for them, and run them only if they have the viewer's interest. Some viewers rarely run more than a single flow; others often do.

THE FLOWS IN BASIC TIR

In Basic TIR, the instructions for the flows differ only on the INC step. As mentioned earlier, you do not need an instruction in order to find an incident to run with Basic TIR. The viewer will give it to you during the assessment phase. But after you have completed TIR on that incident, it can be a good idea to check other "live" flows. If the first incident run was clearly inflow, you would then proceed as above and check outflow, crossflow, and reflexive flow in sequence. Sometimes inflow and reflexive flow describe the same incidents, and sometimes other flows are similarly "fused". If that's the case, you wouldn't run the same incident twice. If you do not know, or cannot be sure, which flow or flows a given incident represented to your client, just ask him/her. Usually it will be obvious.

When you are about to check another flow, make sure the viewer is oriented to the original incident, the one (s)he ran first. If the viewer started with an incident of being mugged and you have just discharged that one in one session, when you come into the next session, you might say something like: "Do you recall the incident we ran last session?" If (s)he does not, simply reorient to it. Once (s)he knows which incident you are talking about, ask: "Is there a time when you caused another to have an experience similar to that one?"* If the viewer comes up with one that seems to be charged and that has his/her interest, address it just as you did the original incident. Then, when the outflow incident is discharged, you can check, and, if necessary, discharge the crossflow and reflexive flow. Wordings for the flows in Basic TIR are as follows:

Inflow	*"Is there a time when another caused you to have an experience similar to that one?"***
Outflow	*"Is there a time when you caused another to have an experience similar to that one?"*
Crossflow	*"Is there a time when others caused others to have an experience similar to that one?"*
Reflexive flow	*"Is there a time when you caused yourself to have an experience similar to that one?"*

Each time, you have to reorient the viewer to the original incident so that (s)he knows what you mean when you say, "that one". The EI instruction remains the same for all flows, *"Is there an earlier similar incident?"*

---

* Note that merely asking that question in the wrong tone of voice can instantly render the space unsafe for your client. Be careful to ask in a nonaccusatory way. A variation you might wish to use is, *"Is there a time when you* might have *caused another...."* Whichever you use, be consistent.

** You would use this inflow question only if the original incident—the first one you addressed—was not an inflow incident.

THE FLOWS IN THEMATIC TIR

In Thematic TIR, you start out with *"Find an incident containing* [theme]." Observe that the direction of flow is not specified in this instruction. You will have to judge what the flow is from how the viewer describes the incident. When you get to the EI instruction, you will want to ask for the proper flow. The questions for checking the INC step on the different flows are:

Inflow　　　　　*"Is there an incident that could have caused you to have* [theme—e.g., a feeling of pure panic]*?"*

Outflow　　　　*"Is there a time when you caused another to have* [theme]*?"*

Crossflow　　　*"Is there a time when others caused others to have* [theme]*?"*

Reflexive flow　*"Is there a time when you caused yourself to have* [theme]*?"*

The corresponding EI instructions are:

Inflow　　　　　*"Is there an earlier incident that could have caused you to have* [theme]*?"*

Outflow　　　　*"Is there an earlier time when you caused another to have* [theme]*?"*

Crossflow　　　*"Is there an earlier time when others caused others to have* [theme]*?"*

Reflexive flow　*"Is there an earlier time when you caused yourself to have* [theme]*?"*

UNBLOCKING

8

New subject: a lady close to sixty years old, petite ... someone who's spent most of her life as a social worker, rape and crisis counselor, homeless shelter operator, family abuse counselor—a person who, herself, was sexually and verbally abused. Her mother had committed suicide, two marriages ended in divorce, and her last husband also committed suicide. He was a man who had lived a sham, lived an untrue life, assumed a lifestyle and identity and activities that were all lies. When his money ran out and he was no longer able to continue that lie, he put a shotgun in his mouth and blew his head off. She found him, still hanging on the shotgun.

When I met her, she had received professional counseling for over 18 months. She had just taken a part time job as a nursing assistant and was in the process of losing her home, having run out of all savings, down to nothing. The insurance money was spent, and she was basically being forced back out of the home and onto the street to survive or to commit suicide herself, an act she had considered.

That's when I entered the picture, again through a mutual friend, a person I'd worked with that she knew. I started working with her. At the time, she had very acute arthritis in her hands—the skin drawn very tightly over the knuckles, over the fingers, over the bones. It didn't go with the rest of her at all. She had basically no flexibility in any of her fingers. We worked through the last suicide, and in the process, I recall her agonizing over the fact that the sheriff and the people who had investigated on that morning had told her not to wash her hands, and had basically accused her of assisting him to commit suicide. (Obviously, they were looking at the paraffin test for residual gunpowder on her hands.) She was not involved, and she was fully acquitted very quickly, but ... a strange thing: at no time, through all of that process, did they ever come back to her and tell her that she could wash her hands now.

Within ten minutes of completing our first session, she got up, went to the kitchen sink, took a bar of soap, and started scrubbing her hands, looking at me—crying, and laughing—and said, "My God, I can wash my hands again for the first time in two years."

Quite an impact on "the Wildcat." He almost lost it!

Several sessions later, she had a major realization concerning her sexual abuser, and this was coupled to her having been raised as a young lady on a farm, where she had also been sexually abused. When it went all the way back, she had a very definite realization that it was not her fault. She ended up going back to her own counselor, helping him through a couple of sessions, becoming one of his case studies—to be presented during a national meeting. Yet she withheld from that counselor the fact that she had realized where her problems had been rooted, and the case presentation turned into one in which, during a seminar, her counselor's peers attempted to tell him where he had gone wrong, what he should have done, how he might have been able to get to the bottom of the issue had he used different techniques ... and they used it as a problem solving seminar. The lady's attitude, when she heard about it, was "Let them work it out. I did."

She, today, is very happy doing what she is doing. She is working full time and has picked up—through her use of TIR—some techniques that she has incorporated into her own case load. She is, in fact, in charge of her life and, in her words, "quite happy".

TIR is one of the more potent tools among the myriad applications that have derived to date from metapsychology, but it is far from being the only one, and though robust, and effective in addressing and resolving a large number of presenting conditions, it is by no means simply a "stand-alone" technique. For one thing, TIR does not lend itself well to addressing every kind of emotionally charged issue that a client might elect to bring up. There are other tools that cover most of the gaps, however, and one of the most broadly useful of these is called "Unblocking".

A REPETITIVE PROCEDURE

Unblocking is a technique that makes use of repetition as a means of allowing a client to examine an item or issue from a number of viewpoints which (s)he may, in effect, have "blocked" comprehension. We block our awareness (or permit it to be blocked) in various ways and for various reasons. We may wish, for instance, to feel more comfortable about an unpleasant situation, and so *suppress* some feeling or thought we might otherwise have about it. Or perhaps, fearing to offend another, we *invalidate* some obvious indication that the other has made a serious *mistake*. In general, we prevent our own awareness by "blocking" it through the use of one or another sort of personal avoidance strategy. We may allow our convictions to be subsumed by the *suggestions* of an authority; we may be *cautious about, conceal,* or *falsify* information or a perception that troubles us. Whatever blocks we adopt, though, the net effect of our failure to examine them, of course, is not really to protect us as we would wish, but to lessen our ability to confront—and thus become able to resolve—whatever is troubling us.

In making use of the Unblocking procedure, you will be directing your client to inspect a number of such blocks repetitively, one at a time. The use of repetitive questions encourages continuous and close inspection and so leads to increased awareness. But as it is unlikely that an inexperienced viewer will ever before have had the same question asked of him/her more than once, you will need to explain your reasons for doing it before you begin. Depending on the client's level of sophistication, your explanation may be very brief, or may need to be fairly detailed.

Repetitive procedures such as Unblocking are one of the cornerstones of viewing. As Gerbode has observed, repetition is useful not only for developing skills and acquiring or changing habits but for achieving a thorough and penetrating awareness of a particular topic. If insufficiently respectful of the communication skills that need to be employed in the administration of these procedures, however, or of the Rules of Facilitation (especially numbers six and ten), a facilitator may feel it is unnatural and uncomfortable to repeat precisely the same question or instruction each time, and so will tend to vary it during a procedure. If a viewer were troubled by a situation involving his son, for example, and such a facilitator were to attempt to address this concern with Unblocking, instead of simply and quite literally repeating the same question until the viewer had run out of answers, the facilitator would feel compelled to vary the wording from time to time. Instead of just, "Regarding your son, has anything been misunderstood," the facilitator might be inclined to ask, "Is there anything you haven't understood concerning your son?" and then "Have there been any misunderstandings regarding your son?" and then "Have you misunderstood anything about your son?" and then "What else have you misunderstood about that subject?" and even, "Find something else you've failed to grasp regarding your son."

Since each of these questions asks the viewer essentially the same thing, why should it make any difference whether we keep to the same wording, or vary it? The answer lies in the Rules of Facilitation and in the basic mechanics of viewing. Two of the Rules of Facilitation are particularly apropos in this case:

> Rule 6. Be interest*ed*, not interest*ing*.
> Rule 10. Act predictably.

As we have suggested repeatedly, it is important that the actions of the therapist and the mechanics of the session fade into the background and become transparent, so that the client can place his/her full attention on what (s)he, as the viewer, is doing. And repetition reduces distraction.

> It is a fact of human nature that something repetitive and *unchanging* in the environment (like a dripping faucet or a ticking clock) tends to become invisible. Things that *change* come into the foreground and they naturally attract attention. Deliberately becoming uninteresting is somewhat difficult for most of us because it goes against normal social practice. In normal conversation and in writing, we do vary our words because we *wish* to be interesting, to be in the listener's "foreground" so as to attract the attention needed to get our viewpoint across. In a world of interesting things and people, we learn to try to be more different and unusual than the competition, so that we will be noticed. But in a viewing session, we are *not* trying to get our point of view across to the viewer. Quite the contrary, in fact. We want the viewer to find his/her *own* point of view, so we want to make ourselves and the viewing procedure itself uninteresting. Adhering to a single wording of a viewing instruction helps accomplish this aim. [13b]

WHEN TO USE UNBLOCKING

You can apply Unblocking successfully to a great many emotionally charged areas in a viewer's life where TIR would be less workable or appropriate. Often, as mentioned below, you can use it to prepare a viewer to run TIR. You will find it to be especially useful for cooling off situations that exist for him/her in or close to the present moment. In TIR, and particularly Basic TIR, you will typically be asking your viewer to focus on past, heavily charged incidents. Sometimes, however, the viewer's attention will be so fixed on a person or event close to the present or of such immediate concern to him/her that (s)he won't be able to focus on what (s)he needs to look at in TIR until you have handled the immediate problem. If (s)he knows his/her car is on fire in the parking lot, (s)he isn't going to have much attention available for reducing past traumas until the fire is out.

Unblocking won't put out a fire in the parking lot, but it can produce rapid and often remarkable results when you use it to address specific people or situations on which your viewer's attention is fixed. Such fixations might include: her husband, his wife, his daughter, her job (or losing it), the burglary of her house, his marriage, her supervisor, her parents, his son, computers, being disorganized, her demotion, his last therapist, the hospital. Each and every one of those topics and a host of others have proven to be suitable grist for the mill of Unblocking.

If you have clients who have had earlier therapeutic experiences prior to coming to you for help, sometimes, even frequently, perhaps, such experiences will not always have been pleasant, and your client will have emotional charge connected with therapy itself. Unfortunately, many therapists tend to violate the Rules of Facilitation to a degree that disturbs or alienates a significant percentage of their clients. This may happen perhaps most often and most damagingly in overburdened institutional settings. At any rate, questions designed to uncover any such experiences should be a regular part of any intake interview, because any client of yours who has previously undergone therapy by which (s)he felt harmed rather than helped is likely to begin his/her work with you by being extremely wary of you and your intentions. The viewer may well identify you, consciously or unconsciously, as being the same as "that other shrink", or "those bastards at the hospital". You may have real trouble in getting him/her to differentiate between what you are about to do with him/her, and what they—as the client perceived it—did (or attempted to do) to him/her. In such a case, begin by using the Unblocking procedure to address "your previous experience(s) with therapy", or "your sessions with the crisis counselor", or "the hospital", or whatever fits. At a minimum, the end point will involve your being thoroughly differentiated in the mind of your client from earlier therapists, and able to go on to TIR (or whatever else you plan to do) with a clean slate.

HOW TO DO UNBLOCKING

As we noted above, the Unblocking list which follows is made up of a number of common mental blocks. Most of the questions on the Unblocking lists can be answered with reference to more than just one flow (e.g., "Yes, she suppressed me by...", "I suppressed her when I ...", "He suppressed my father", "I suppressed my thoughts", and so forth). Encourage your client to consider any and all of them that could be appropriate when looking for instances of the various blocks. This will open up areas of charge in some clients at which it might not otherwise occur to them to look. Addressing each line repetitively with your client and permitting him/her to communicate about it—and simply to have the communications acknowledged—causes charge to be reduced and the stimulation removed from the area you are addressing.

Make it clear to your client that:

- (S)he will have as many opportunities as desired to answer a given question.
- You only want one answer each time you ask the question and not every answer (s)he might think of all at once.
- You will repeat the question as many times as (s)he has answers to it.

The variation of the Unblocking list that we provide in this chapter consists of 24 blocks. As with TIR and any other viewing procedure, the first step is to make sure that your client understands his/her role in running the procedure, and that (s)he may include any "flow" in the answers that a given question permits. Also, let the client know that you expect him/her to include some data in each answer, beyond just saying, "Yes". As always, consult your client's interest before selecting a topic to run.

Suppose, for instance, that you attempt to address a major childhood issue of your client's with TIR, but discover that his/her interest and concern is tightly focused on immediate difficulties having to do with his supervisor at work. (The supervisor, then, would be the "car on fire in the parking lot".) Because you are unable to direct his/her attention easily to the trauma that (s)he originally came to you to handle, your first job becomes one of handling the emotional charge connected with the supervisor. Once you have a topic to address—"your supervisor", in this instance—you use it as a prefix to each of the items ("blocks") on the Unblocking list. In this case, you would phrase your question something like this, "Regarding your supervisor, is there any-thing that has been ____?", filling in the blank with each of the blocks on the Unblocking list in sequence, beginning with the first one, suppressed.

If your client tells you (s)he is not interested in or has no further answers to a particular block, then simply acknowledge this, leave that block, and go on to the next. As in any facilitation, be sure to acknowledge each and every answer as your viewer gives it to you. Pursue each block by asking the appropriate question *repetitively*. Take each block on the list to some sort of end point, though not necessarily a major one. Perhaps the viewer has a little flash of insight, "I wonder if that might not be why..." Further, the client says (with congruent indicators) that (s)he feels a little better. Or (s)he simply runs out of answers or loses interest in that block. You then go on to the next block on the list—"invalidated"—and ask, "Regarding your job (or your wife, or whatever topic you are addressing), has anything or anyone been invalidated?" You then repeat that question until you reach another minor end point or your client runs out of answers. Continue in this fashion until one of the following occurs:

1. Your client reaches a significant end point or some kind of success in the area being addressed—one that (s)he is clearly happy about.*
2. You have completed the list of blocks.
3. The viewer feels that there is nothing more (s)he needs to handle on the topic you have been Unblocking.

Sometimes, in the middle of Unblocking, something will come up in the way of a major disturbance for the client, some incident or event that is particularly upsetting to him/her when (s)he encounters it. Usually, you will be able to resolve this successfully by simply continuing to ask the question that triggered the reaction. On occasion, however, you may turn up a heavy disturbance that refuses to go away despite simple repetition of the question that brought it into view. In that case, you may have to handle the disturbance with TIR. Then, after you have completed the TIR, just go back to Unblocking, finish handling the block you were working on, and continue on to the next block. Never leave "unfinished business" in your wake. Unblocking is very simple but also extremely effective in providing a rapid reduction of the triggering effects of environmental stressors. If you plan to use TIR, you might wish to consider using Unblocking on an appropriate subject first with one or more of your clients, so as to get a "feel" for what it is like to operate within the constraints imposed by the Rules of Facilitation and by what we have said about communication while dealing with this simple pattern before launching into the relatively more complex and demanding TIR procedure.

---

* Be prepared for the possibility that this may happen quite early on in the list, particularly with an experienced viewer. Do not continue the list—or any other viewing procedure—beyond its end point.

THE UNBLOCKING LIST

Regarding (subject) ...

1. Is there anything* that has been suppressed? [prevented from being seen/heard/felt (by oneself or by someone or something else); held down; kept under]**
2. Is there anything that has been invalidated? [made wrong; criticized; belittled]
3. Is there anything that has been evaluated? [judged; assessed]
4. Is there anything that you have been cautious about? [wary of; careful about]
5. Is there anything that has been resisted? [fought against; tried not to do]
6. Is there anything that hasn't been revealed? [made known; uncovered]
7. Is there anything that you have been worried about? [anxious about; troubled by]
8. Is there anything that has been changed? [altered; moved]
9. Has there been a mistake? [error; misjudgment]
10. Has there been a failure? [something disappointing; a loss]
11. Has anything not been acknowledged? [made nothing of; not given credit]
12. Has there been a protest? [disagreement; objection]
13. Is there anything that has been avoided? [withdrawn from; retreated/distanced from]
14. Is there anything that has been ignored? [disregarded; dismissed]
15. Is there anything that has been withheld? [kept from; not given/offered to; hidden]
16. Has anyone made a suggestion? [advised; proposed]
17. Has anyone felt strongly about something? [asserted anything]
18. Has anyone been blamed for something? [accused; held responsible for]
19. Is there anything that has been agreed with? [cooperated with; gone along with]
20. Is there anything that has been disagreed with? [argued with; rejected]

---

* As appropriate, you may wish to add "or anyone" to some of these questions.
** Alternative terms such as those provided in brackets may communicate better to a given client than the one given in the body of the question. Choose the one that you feel will best communicate to a given client, and once chosen, do not vary it.

21. Is there anything that has been enforced? [forced on anyone; made to accept]
22. Is there anything that has been decided? [chosen; elected]
23. Has anything been achieved? [finished; accomplished]
24. Is there anything that has been overlooked? [not noticed; forgotten about]

Remember that your client may reach an end point on this list well before reaching the end of the list itself, and be prepared to stop if and when that happens; do not feel that you must ask every question.

A point to bear in mind, too, is that your own knowledge of a particular client may suggest other blocks that you might want to add to the list to check. The list above will produce change, relief, and insights in a large majority of cases, but it is neither sacred nor inviolate, and you might wish to expand it on occasion. If you have reason to think that your client has experienced rejection in the part of his/her life that you plan to address—rejection of him/herself or his/her ideas or contributions—you might, for example, add "Has anything or anyone been rejected?" to the list before you assess it. Whenever you make that sort of case-specific alteration to this or any other viewing procedure, however, be certain that any question or instruction that you have constructed with the aid of privileged knowledge does not come across to your client/viewer as accusatory in any way. It will be best, as suggested earlier, if you present such items somewhere in the middle of the list as simply another block, and be quite willing to accept an answer that does not fit with your own (unshared!) evaluation of the situation your client is viewing.

We may carefully have crafted a question in order to give our client the opportunity to look at, talk about, and resolve an issue that we, in our infinite wisdom, have decided is the very core of the difficulties in the area being addressed. In the strictly client-centered context that this work is done in, however, we must have nothing invested in the answer to the question. If the viewer says, "No, I don't think so" to such a question, we acknowledge gracefully and go on to the next question.

Ultimately, the only wisdom that counts in the sort of session we are describing in this text, is that of the client.

CLIENT FOCUS

9

New subject: a Vietnam combat vet, a skilled technician, within six months of being able to retire ... diagnosed with a nervous breakdown. He came to me asking, "How do I get back into the federal system now that I have bailed out of it? Is there any way I can get back in?"

We went through a few alternatives, and then I gave him a short session that had an outstanding result. We then went through five of six more sessions. They started out, oh, two, two and a half hours a shot ... ended up fifteen-twenty minutes a session. He finally came to realize that a set of common circumstances were involved in the work site of his last job where he'd finally just gotten to a point where he could not work, could not concentrate, could not sleep, did not eat, went back on the bottle.... All of those things had common leads back to Vietnam and what he had done there. He saw. He drew the parallels between them. He had the realizations. And the last I heard from him, two months ago, he was back with his old organization ... everyone was happy to have him back ... and he was well on his way to passing his probation period. He's off and running. He did well....

EMPOWERMENT

Viewing in general and TIR in particular is designed to empower the client, and it is critically important that we permit that to happen, despite the many invitations we may receive as therapists to do our clients' work for them, thus incurring their dependence: "What do you think it means when I _____,

Doctor?" "Am I spending too much time worrying about my husband?" "Do you think I should spend more time working on my mother?" "Could that actually have happened?" "Am I getting better?" The answers to any and all such questions, if tendered by the facilitator, will disempower the viewer, whose proper role in viewing involves becoming able to make all such determinations with confidence and without outside "assistance".

Yet at the same time, clients do have valid questions, and we as their therapists or facilitators may and often do have the knowledge that can help them. Clients often seek our advice to help them cope with a great variety of issues such as a seemingly precocious, overactive, and sexually aggressive child; a woman who wants to be told what she should do about her spouse's drinking problem; or a man whose entire life seems to be a logistical nightmare and he asks us for help in sorting it out.

The question then arises: how can you attach as much significance to the Rules of Facilitation as we have earlier suggested that you must* and at the same time continue to maintain the supportive role you are almost certainly required to play from time to time as therapist?

We can and should perhaps reverse the question as well, how can you make use of your hard-won knowledge and skills as a supportive therapist without running afoul of those same Rules? If followed assiduously, the Rules would seem to prohibit your use of an impressively large number of valuable and commonly employed tools of the therapist's trade. One can hardly give advice without evaluation, for instance, and counsel generally involves validation, interpretation, and even invalidation—the use of any one of which violates the Rules of Facilitation. So while we believe it possible that the amount of advice and counsel that one's clients require may be significantly—even vastly—less than one might have imagined prior to making use of TIR and Unblocking, still, there certainly remains a need for those tools and the knowledge and expertise that they require. But their use in conjunction with TIR will cause the latter to fall far short of its potential.

What to do?

That is—or soon becomes—an important question for any therapist whose interest in making use of TIR or Unblocking** is sufficiently robust to cause him/her to take the protocols seriously and thus to adhere in session to all the tenets described in this chapter and the last. On the one hand, if

---

* Must, that is, in order to achieve the full results that TIR and Unblocking are capable of producing.

** Or any other among the hundreds of procedures that currently constitute the myriad applications of metapsychology.

your interest in your profession has ever flagged, you are likely to find it rejuvenated when you experience the power of the tools you will have introduced to your work. On the other hand, you will encounter scenarios not unlike the following: in mid-session, addressing a mugging, your client suddenly tells you ("originates") that she has decided to divorce her husband and desperately needs advice on how to handle various of the consequences she can foresee.

Again, what to do? As a TIR facilitator, you are being told to keep the focus on the item being addressed and the procedure being used, but as a therapist, you may also recognize that your client's question is deserving of supportive discussion of a sort that the TIR protocols would seem to discourage, if not actively to prevent. If the TIR is to bring about full resolution, then you, the facilitator, though you certainly care and are interested, must remain to a significant degree detached, and your communication austere. Yet it will be important for you, the therapist, to be able to be supportive on occasion as well.

INTEGRATING TIR INTO TRADITIONAL PSYCHOTHERAPY

Until very recently, the question of how to integrate the two quite different modes or roles—therapist and facilitator—had not really been addressed at all, with the result that some less-than-wholly felicitous adaptations occurred in various practices. Helen Burgess, a gifted facilitator and long-time friend and professional associate of Gerbode and French, is the first we are aware of to have spoken clearly, albeit informally, to a need for clarification of this area: "The viewing mode becomes ineffective when mixed with the support role [and vice versa], and ideally it should come to be perceived as part of the therapist/client relationship rather than as simply part of the way an isolated technique [such as TIR or Unblocking] is administered" (e-mail correspondence with French, 1997). Burgess believes that the supportive role of the therapist is what permits a therapeutic relationship to be built with a client. She suggests, however, that if a therapist—newly impressed with the power to be found in viewing procedures such as TIR whose protocols demand strict adherence to the Communication Exercises and the Rules of Facilitation—were to attempt to relate to a client solely on the basis of those parameters, (s)he would find him/herself unable to build that kind of relationship. Nor could (s)he offer the kind of support the client sometimes truly needs. Virtually by definition, the viewing modality does not include a relationship-building function. If the therapist remains solely in a supportive role, however, and does not permit clients to view as well—and thus to be granted full responsibility for their own progress in a given area, such as recovery from emotional trauma—then clients are all too likely to become dependent on the therapist, looking to the latter to provide answers to questions that no therapist should attempt to answer for a client who is capable of coming up with his/her own answers.

The client often needs—and, we would maintain, is able—to look to and for him/herself to be able to face the pain, and then to decide what to do about it. And the viewing function, where pure client-centered work prevails, is the best modus operandi for such work. So there is a need for both support and viewing, but the two have often in practice been combined; when that happens, each becomes less effective.

Typically, the closest that therapists and lay facilitators have come to handling the problem effectively is to make a policy of explaining the difference between the two functions to new clients. That is certainly a valid and important thing to do. But Burgess points out that there is something more that should be done as well. Whenever she has found herself "diluting the viewing model" with inappropriately supportive efforts to respond "helpfully" to a viewer's originations, it has been because she knew that viewing alone was not adequate (to handle, for example, the effects of having a codependent relationship with an alcoholic), yet had not worked out a way of alternating gracefully and effectively between the two modalities.

Burgess now addresses the problem by carefully defining the different roles before beginning work with a client, making sure that the client clearly understands that the two "hats" can and, as required, will both be worn, but never at the same time. In brief, she explains that when acting as facilitator, her job will be solely to provide a structure that the client can use to conduct his/her *own* investigation into, and resolution of, a high percentage of the issues (s)he has come to her wishing to handle.* She goes over the Rules of Facilitation with the client and explains that as facilitator, she will never discuss, or suggest solutions to, any issue the client may be dealing with as a viewer, but that if the client should feel the need for a response from or dialogue with her in her support role regarding any subject of concern, (s)he will have ample opportunity to do so outside of the context of viewing, both

---

* Just how high that percentage will or can be depends on a number of factors, the most important being, of course, the number and type of issues with which the client presents.

before the start and after the close of a viewing session,* and at a time the client requests one or more sessions of pure consultation or support other than viewing.

Before formally starting a session of viewing, she asks every client (never varying the question), "Is there anything you wish to talk to me about before we begin the [viewing] session?" After closing the session, she asks no question, but makes it clear that she is available within reason should the client wish to discuss the formal session or any other issues. She makes no comments whatsoever about the session, of course, nor about any material addressed in it, and she makes it clear that she never will, unless the client brings it up and requests a dialogue outside of viewing.

"My husband hit me again last night. Maybe I really should leave him and go to a shelter, but...." Such a concern would be difficult to address in the pure viewing mode without reducing the efficacy of viewing. If, however, this client clearly understands the two different functions a practitioner can fulfill in a session and when they each will occur, she can choose to bring up the beating by her husband in either the viewing or the support mode, knowing that the therapist/facilitator will address it accordingly—with consultation, advice, and perhaps referrals while in "support mode" and with the tools discussed earlier for handling originations while in the viewing mode.

If the distinction between the two modalities has not been made clear, support functions invariably bleed into the viewing approach and viewing functions are attempted while in the support mode; neither modality produces the results that it could; and the client is much more likely to remain dependent and disenfranchised.

Throughout this book, our comments and observations concern primarily the viewing mode, and we have proceeded on the assumption that you are already familiar and comfortable otherwise with playing a support role for your clients. As a facilitator, then, your work should not involve doing anything whatsoever for the viewer other than directing the session. Much more often than not, you will find (if you have not already) that the most productive, dramatic, and life-changing cognitive shifts occur when clients have had their own realizations and not yours. In sum, when acting as facilitator, don't do anything that substitutes for or interferes with your

---

* Viewing sessions should be begun and ended formally by the therapist/facilitator, so that the client knows when the facilitator is governed by the Rules of Facilitation. Thus there is always a period of time in a session, both before and after that formal announcement, during which consultation and support can occur if necessary.

client's exercise of his/her own powers and perception. As suggested earlier, this would include telling a viewer:

1. What (s)he is seeing
2. What it means
3. How (s)he should direct his/her life
4. That (s)he is wrong
5. That (s)he is right.

In doing either of the first two, you are interpreting for the viewer. If you succumb to the temptations of numbers three, four, and five, you are evaluating—and, in the case of number four, invalidating—the person or his/her ideas. The fifth is that form of evaluation we call validation, of course. As we have noted elsewhere, though seeming perhaps at first blush to be an excellent thing to do, it will not help you as a facilitator in your efforts to empower your client.

So how do we truly integrate TIR and related work into more traditional psychotherapy? There are as many models of psychotherapy as there are psychotherapists who practice them. These days, psychotherapy ranges from vocational counseling to genetic counseling; from marriage and family therapy to group counseling; and from individual counseling to multifamily therapy. Each has its own methodologies and its own techniques brought into the session by the unique entity that is the therapist.

As we have already seen, there are a great many traditional psychotherapeutic models into which TIR cannot easily fit. The approach resists Procrustean efforts to force it into any mold formed around the idea that the client's job is pretty much just to talk to the psychotherapist, whose job it is in turn to interpret content so the client has a better understanding of the process that requires change. From this we could infer that the clients probably talk between 50 and 75 percent of a session while the therapist talks 25 to 50 percent of the time. This is the psychoanalytic legacy of Freud which persists today in most modern psychotherapeutic models, and it is antithetical to the effective use of TIR or any other form of viewing.

As you may have realized by this point, however, TIR is client-focused [18] to such a degree that in a typical TIR session, more than 90 percent of the words spoken will be said by the client, and fewer than ten by the facilitator/therapist. Further, TIR stresses the nonparticipation of the facilitator. As a result, TIR can fit traditional psychotherapy as a unique therapeutic intervention. Unique in that, as an intervention, a single use of it will most likely take up an entire session and will be a new experience for the client unfamiliar with viewing.

French is fond of telling TIR trainees that the best facilitators can often be those who are not trained as therapists. This is because the nontherapist seems so much more easily to be able to resist the urge to intervene than does the trained interventionist. It is exactly these interventionist urges that must be resisted. Because philosophically, TIR is so close to those schools of psychotherapy that advocate client- rather than therapist-initiated change, the therapist coming from a more client-focused background will tend, logically, to be more successful when using TIR.

Although most therapeutic models recognize that the impetus for change lies with the client, methods of achieving this change are to be found in abundance, and vary dramatically. Looking only within the sphere of marriage and family therapy, for example, there are volumes [16, 17] that reference therapeutic models as numerous and disparate as behavioral family therapy, contextual family therapy, family systems therapy, functional family therapy, interactional family therapy, Milan systemic family therapy, structural family therapy, strategic family therapy, and symbolic-experimental family therapy—to name only a representative sample. Each of these models embodies specific methodologies and techniques which dictate how change occurs.

Two examples from the marriage and family therapy models we have listed above may serve as illustrations for determining which therapeutic models might meld with TIR from a philosophical perspective. Strategic family therapy is a communication therapy [28]. In making use of it, the therapist is charged with originating what happens during the therapy session and is responsible for arranging a specific approach for the difficulties presented. Stanton [28, p. 361] writes, "Strategic therapists take responsibility for directly influencing people [clients]." On the other hand, Milan systemic family therapy charges the therapist with "neutrality" [6, p. 328]. This admonition compels the practitioner to avoid adopting any position, positive or negative, regarding the specific behavioral outcome of therapy.

Thus, although both strategic family therapy and Milan systemic family therapy achieve change for the clients, the nondirective Milan model is more nearly philosophically consistent with TIR. That being the case, we might expect that the Milan family therapist would find training in TIR and related techniques to be easier—and the integration of the tools into his practice less jarring—than might the strategic family therapist. However, it should be noted that regardless of the therapeutic bias of the therapist-to-become-facilitator, adherence to the dictates set out in this text should result in successful TIR facilitation as an intervention technique.

As noted earlier, then, the roles of therapist/supporter and of facilitator are radically different; if each is used in its proper place, however, they can be superb complements to one another. Do not mix the two, however, and recall always, when acting as facilitator, that you must not do anything that interferes with or—worse—substitutes for your client's exercise of his/her own wisdom, insight, powers, and perception.

CONTRAINDICATIONS AND CORRECTIONS **10**

Another guy: a graduate student, male, the son of a friend. I watched him go through most of high school and college; some of the normal trials and tribulations as he interacted with members of the opposite sex. He's one of those people with a gift for dealing with people ... liked by everyone who knows him ... never had a problem getting dates with the girls. But then, in graduate school, he fell deeply in love with a girl whom he wanted to marry. They discussed it, planned how it would happen ... and then it all unraveled, and very unpleasantly.

Well, falling off the deep end ("That's all that I deserve"), he turned into a real wild person. He almost flunked out of school ... withdrew from several courses ... was suspended briefly ... went back to school ... and was not doing very well at all. Not interacting well with people as he always had before ... working part time ... going to the bars and raising six kinds of sand almost full time. Wasn't a whole lot of time for studies.

He'd heard about what I was doing [with TIR] from his dad, and one day he came to me asked if maybe I could "try that stuff" with him. Within two weeks time—during which, as I recall, we had four or five sessions—he crawled out of the bars, picked up his books, and went back to studying. He's now graduated, with an MBA, and working hard in a very good job. He has read just about everything that he can get his hands on that has to do with TIR. He's extremely interested in learning all of the processes and procedures, and would like to pick it up.....

Again, he was an individual who was heading down the wrong track, knew he was heading down the wrong track, needed a "tour guide" to turn him around, got one ... and turned around. He's doing great!

And I suspect that's about enough rambling into this little machine, so before too long goes past, I will get the tape in the mail. One of these days, I'd like to learn more about this stuff myself. I realize that in TIR, I've got just a little piece of it....

CONTRAINDICATIONS

This chapter addresses situations that mitigate against one's use of TIR with a client, and provides two short lists of questions/instructions that you can use—in the first instance, to "repair" a TIR session that has gone off the rails; in the second, to destimulate a client who has been triggered by the session focus but whom you have simply not been able to bring to an end point.

TIR is a potent tool, and it works well when used to address a very broad spectrum of both clients and conditions, but there are certainly factors which, when present, render it a poor form of address to any issue. The use of TIR is contraindicated when any of the following conditions exist:

1. The client is in session for reasons not his/her own.
2. The client is significantly distracted by immediate concerns better suited to address by other means.
3. The client is currently feeling the effects of mind-altering drugs.
4. The client is too young for the formal procedure.
5. The client carries an incompatible diagnosis.
6. The facilitator is poorly trained and insufficiently respectful of the contextual requirements of viewing in general and TIR in particular.

In Session for the Wrong Reasons

The 11th Rule of Facilitation states, "Never attempt a session with a client who is unwilling or protesting." Possibly the easiest way to violate that rule is to take on a client who has been sent to you by the courts—or whose spouse or employer has insisted that (s)he get "help"—without first making sure that (s)he has, or can find, at least one reason for being in session with you that is entirely valid in his/her own estimation.

That does not mean that you cannot help such a client—only that in order to have any hope of being able to do so, you will first need to get into good communication with him/her. That will not happen unless and until you and (s)he have openly discussed the fact of having come to you under protest, and you have acknowledged the futility of asking, let alone demanding, change of anyone under such conditions. Once you have accomplished that step, however, your client will have a level of trust and belief in you that was previously lacking, and you may very well be able to help find a reason to proceed that (s)he finds valid—some aspect of his/her life that is important to *him/her* to change.

Distractions

We've mentioned this point earlier. It's the "car on fire in the parking lot." When your client has an immediate concern (one rooted in the present) that is sufficiently distracting, TIR will not work. You will need to take up and destimulate the concern before your client will have enough free attention available to him/her to address past events. It is important to be aware that this condition will not always be an obvious one. If your client is inclined towards propitiation or regards you too readily as being the authority in the room, (s)he may very well cooperatively take up a theme or incident with TIR when you suggest it, even if (s)he has too much else on his/her mind to do well with the procedure. Thus, before starting a TIR session, you will be well advised to ask your client directly if (s)he has her attention on any sort of upsetting situation, problem, or undelivered (unspoken) communication.

Distractions are almost always subsumed under one of three headings: upsets, problems, or things that the client has attention on not having communicated. A fourth—a thing the client may have done that (s)he is feeling guilty about—is sometimes present as well, and you can check for it if you suspect that it might be. A word of warning concerning this last, however, if you have earlier either violated the Rules of Facilitation to any significant degree, or failed to handle session communication as we have said that you will need to, it is highly unlikely that your client will feel sufficiently safe with you to admit to wrongdoings as such. You must ask the question in a wholly nonaccusatory fashion ("Do you have attention on anything you've done that you wish you hadn't?" for example, or "Have you done something you felt was wrong?" and *not*, "Have you done something wrong?"), and when your client has answered, of course, do not attempt to "work through" or in any other way address whatever your client has told you. Simply acknowledge your client's communication. The power of that simple acknowledgment to resolve the guilt (and to enable the client to avoid the behavior in the future!) may well astonish you.*

Finally, recalling our admonitions concerning closing and putting away every "box" you open before opening another, always ask about each of those potential distractions as separate questions.

Drugs

There has not been any research we can find on the effectiveness of TIR on subjects under the influence of drugs, but a wealth of anecdotal evidence suggests strongly that the following general statements are accurate:

1. Clients carrying a dual diagnosis involving drugs or alcohol do not do well with TIR and, therefore, it should not be attempted with them.
2. Neither lithium nor selective serotonin reuptake inhibitors (SSRIs) seem to interfere with TIR and the viewing procedure.

The following observations from a viewer concerning the experience of mixing an SSRI with TIR are consistent with the our experience:

> I recently experienced a course of Traumatic Incident Reduction (TIR)....
> The results in less than one week were dramatic. I feel that most of the
> core issues that psychotherapy or medication could never touch were
> truly *resolved*. For good. I was on the SSRI Paxil while I undertook this
> therapy, but had not been on it long enough for it to have relieved my
> depression, suffering, pain, and anxiety, as well as other disorders.** I
> have never had a remission of depression and related feelings happen so
> completely and so nearly instantaneously. The fact that I was on Paxil
> may have helped me to concentrate better on the processes of the therapy,
> but my honest opinion is that TIR would have been successful whether
> I was on medication or not, and that the medication really neither
> augmented or detracted from its effectiveness.

---

* The Catholic church discovered the healing power of simple (unpunished) confession a long time ago.
** An SSRI, of course, usually requires a number of weeks to "kick in" and reach clinical levels.

Ultimately, it is probable if not certain that any drug that tends to have either a sedative effect* or a tendency to create euphoria** will interfere with the efficacy of TIR at least to some degree. If contraindicated medication is prescribed, however, and your client wishes to attempt the procedure despite understanding that conditions are less than optimal, go ahead with it. The worst that is likely to happen is that the client will not be able to contact the charge in the incident and thus nothing much at all will occur.

Viewer Too Young

Although there are exceptions, preadolescent children are generally not good candidates for either Thematic TIR or formal Basic TIR. They lack the understanding, the motivation, and attention span required.

There is a much simplified version of Basic TIR, however, that does work well in many situations. All it consists of is to ask the child—concernedly, interestedly, and *repeatedly*—to tell you what happened. Be sure to listen carefully to the child's answer, and to acknowledge well following each iteration. Adhere scrupulously to the Rules of Facilitation, just as you would while working with an adult.*** Do not interrupt, validate, invalidate, interpret, evaluate, or overtly sympathize.

The end point you will be looking for with a young child is not quite the same as you might expect in an adult. Children typically will not express or otherwise manifest cognitive shifts, nor will you necessarily be able to bring them to as high a point on the Emotional Scale as you might an adult. Ambivalence or boredom or even perhaps mild antagonism is a reasonable target for a young child who has been deeply fearful or grief stricken, whereas something between contentment and enthusiasm would generally be both desirable and attainable in an adult.

This version of TIR works very well and astonishingly quickly on childhood traumata such as accidents, injuries, nightmares, and incidents containing extreme embarrassment. A parent's use of it with a child who, for instance, has awakened, terrified, from a nightmare, might resemble the following:

---

* This includes many antihistamines, tricyclics (for some people), anxiolytics, and antipsychotic medications such as the phenothiazines.
** Most street/recreational drugs would fit this description.
*** Perhaps in part because children tend to be more self-absorbed than adults, however, a more informal style of both questioning and acknowledging seems to work well with them. See the sample "session" on the next page.

Child:	*[sobbing]* I had a bad dream!
Parent:	Oh, really? Gosh! Well, tell me about it.
Child:	*[sobbing...choking]* There's this horrible monster that ate daddy and it's running after me and...., *[etc.]*
Parent:	Wow...gee, well...tell me about it again.
Child:	*[Crying a bit. Retells, possibly (though not necessarily) with changes.]*
Parent:	I see...gosh, well look...tell me again, OK? *[encouraging]*
Child:	*[some sniffles]* Well, the monster ate daddy and then it came after me....
Parent:	OK, I got it. Hm-mmm! Well, could you tell me again?
Child:	Don't wanna! *[no more sniffles; boredom or mild antagonism]*
Parent:	Oh, OK. Well, I was about to get a glass of warm milk. Want me to get you one?

At this point, the wise parent has dropped the subject of the nightmare and will not mention it again. Typically, the child won't either.

Neither of the present authors has to date attempted working with children on more significant traumata; it may well be that even this abbreviated form of TIR would be too much for some young children in such a case. On the other hand, there are numerous anecdotal reports suggesting that at least some may do very well indeed. Two such reports follow here,* the first concerning a ten-year-old boy, described as presenting with extreme anxiety, not sleeping well, and wanting to be with his parents "all the time", especially at night. When younger, the boy had loved visiting his grandparents an hour's drive from home, but had reached a point of refusing to go there unless his mother and father accompanied him. In addition, he had started wanting to stay away from school. He could give no reason for any of this behavior.

Using thematic TIR, the therapist took up the theme of "being frightened of being alone" (the boy's words) and found an incident that had occurred when the child was about four years old. At that time, he had been sent occasionally to a baby-sitter who, whenever the boy was "naughty", had locked him in a small, dark cupboard under some stairs. In running the incident, the boy discharged a lot of emotion during a session lasting about

* From private correspondence to French from Alex Frater, a TIR-trained therapist in Campbelltown, near Sydney, Australia.

35 minutes. They left it "flat" at the end of that session, but short of a true end point—which they reached in the following session that lasted just 15 minutes. At its end, the boy was laughing about the incident, and his father reported months later that his son's overdependence on his parents and other presenting problems had vanished and not returned.

Another client of that same therapist was a girl, nine years of age, whose bike had been stolen from the new house that she shared with her parents. At the time of the theft, the house had no fence. Subsequent to the incident, she developed day-to-day anxiety, eventually refusing to sleep alone in her own room. Her parents put an extra high fence around the house and even had a heavy lock installed on her windows, to no avail. The girl complained of images of the thieves coming back and ransacking the house and killing her parents and her brother.

Using Basic TIR, the therapist ran that *image** to an end point in less than 25 minutes. In a subsequent session, he checked with the girl for remaining charge and found none. Again, the parents (and the girl) reported no more problems, and the child was sleeping once more "like a baby" in her own room.

Certainly, our own experience suggests that when used to address more nearly quotidian events and situations, the conversational form of TIR which we described above will routinely produce small miracles.

Children tend to run and to reach end points much more quickly than adults, and it is easy to overrun them if you are not observant. Fortunately, they are also inclined to let you know when you have done that—if you have—in no uncertain terms, and a simple acknowledgment accompanied by a quick apology and immediate cessation of the activity is usually all that is necessary to restore or "rehabilitate" a valid end point in a child.

Conditions for Which TIR Is Not the Remedy

There are numerous conditions which are ill-suited for address with TIR. While it would certainly be appropriate to use TIR when dealing with recurring unwanted emotions or attitudes, or with a particular instance of a client's having been traumatized, more generalized problems concerning, for example, communication within a relationship, would not necessarily

---

* Note that they ran—to a good end point—the image of something that had not occurred and was never likely to! This was an excellent and creative use of TIR.

represent a good target for that procedure. Unblocking* would be more appropriate.

TIR is for use with conditions one is troubled by that are the direct or indirect result of past traumata. Although a far higher percentage of such conditions than one might expect seem in fact to have their roots in trauma, not all do.

Incompatible Diagnoses

In order to be able to function effectively as a viewer, one must be able to look at the past from at least a relatively stable platform in the present. Therefore, any diagnosis which suggests the absence of such a viewpoint tends to preclude the use of TIR. Insufficient ego-strength mitigates against its use as does an accurate diagnosis of severe character disorder, significant neurological conditions, or brain damage.

Careful consideration of what the TIR procedure actually requires of a client will suggest who will and will not be an appropriate candidate. Successful viewing demands, at a minimum, sufficient intelligence to understand the procedure and the reasons for its use, a reasonably functional memory, and the ability to apply concentration to a sometimes difficult kind of work. If a diagnosis admits of those, then that diagnosis would not preclude the possibility of using TIR with a client.

Poor Facilitation

When a client's communication is managed as we have earlier described, and the procedure is applied strictly in accordance with the Rules of Facilitation, TIR is an enormously powerful and empowering technique. Assuming that the facilitator has not ignored any of the contraindications above, its failures (when they occur) seem all but inevitably to lie not with any inadequacy of the procedure itself, but with one or another form of misuse of it by the therapist/facilitator. This might include: an end point that was missed and not recovered, one or another violation of the Rules that captured too much of the client's attention for him/her to be able to fully resolve the issue being addressed, or the client's communication mishandled by an overly "caring" facilitator—any number of such errors can interfere with the efficacy of TIR.

---

* Or other, conventional, approaches, or other metapsychological tools beyond the scope of the present work.

Most if not all are avoidable, but some can be quite subtle, and it is much more likely that training or supervision rather than another approach is what is needed by any therapist having significant problems with the use of TIR with clients who have been properly screened.*

CORRECTIONS

Assuming that you have chosen an issue or item to address with TIR or Unblocking that is truly charged and of interest to your client, your client should leave session looking reasonably bright and happy. At the very least, (s)he should be at peace and in a calm frame of mind, with attention on the present and not on the past. On the rare occasions when that does not occur, something has gone wrong which is usually possible to correct. There actually appears to be only a finite number of things that can go wrong in a properly administered TIR session. The most common among them can be found in the short list presented below. If necessary, go over the questions on the list one at a time with your client. Chances are you will be able to find and resolve the problem your client has encountered.

Bearing in mind what we have earlier observed about end points, it is extremely important to pay very close attention to your client's *indicators* from moment to moment during viewing sessions. This is perhaps especially true while working with this list or in any other way trying to sort out something that seems less than optimal during a session. When a client spots or recognizes something that is true or correct or that serves to make sense of some part of his/her mental or emotional environment that has been confused, you will almost always see it in his/her face and manner and tone of voice if you are observant. When you do see it, it is important to recognize it and to determine—if it is not obvious—if something positive has happened that will allow you to call an end to the session or activity you are pursuing.

- *Did we take up something you really were not interested in?* If your client believes that is the case and tells you so with good indicators, simply acknowledge the fact. Some such words as, "Thanks for letting me know that; do you think we need to do anything further about it at this point, then, or does it seem OK to leave it alone?" will usually

---

* We are aware that that comment may appear to be self-serving; it really is not. It is based on extensive evidence observed by the authors and others—including many with no ax to grind—over nearly 15 years of work with the subject.

get a "Yes" answer and increase the number of good indicators in your client, at which point it will be safe (and advisable!) to end the session.

- *Was there, in fact, an earlier, similar incident?* If your client thinks there might have been, find out when it happened and continue and complete TIR from that point.

- *Was the TIR procedure overrun?* [Alternate wording: *Did we go past a point where you felt that (the item/issue being addressed) might have been resolved?*] If so, you will find that you can almost always restore or "recover" the end point by finding out when it occurred, and by having the viewer tell you about it. Solicit details from the viewer until you see good indicators and then end the activity formally by saying something like, "Thanks for letting me know that; we *should* have left it at that point. OK if we do that now?"

- *Were you trying to run TIR in the middle of a distracting upset, worry, or withheld communication?** If yes, then you will need to handle that "car on fire in the parking lot" with Unblocking or another tool before returning to TIR.

- *Might an incident actually have begun earlier?* Find the earlier starting point, and take up the procedure from that point.

REMEDIAL LIST

Should you encounter a viewing session that you have simply not been able to bring to an acceptable end point, you can use the list of instructions given below. If you have taken a workshop or done other training in TIR, you will have access to an instructor with whom you can consult, but your client will leave your office feeling a lot better than (s)he would otherwise if you make use of this list before ending the session. Take the list to a point where the viewer feels better and has his/her attention in the present time. Again, watch your viewer's indicators carefully and be prepared to *stop*, smoothly, when you see significant improvement. It is important to remember that taking your client to a comfortable place by using this list is not the same thing as completing the earlier item that you have had to leave incomplete. In your next session, you will need to ascertain your client's state of mind with regard

---

* A withheld communication is something your client has consciously not told either you or someone else important to him/her ... and it will be something (s)he is not entirely comfortable about.

to the latter, and address as appropriate whatever you find. In using this list, simply preface each of the following with "Remember":

1. ...a time when you shared something with someone.
2. ...a time when you felt real affinity for someone.
3. ...a time when you were in very good communication with someone.
4. ...a time when someone shared something with you.
5. ...a time when someone was in very good communication with you.
6. ...a time when someone really liked you.
7. ...a time when you really liked someone.
8. ...a time when the world seemed very real [agreeable; right] to you.
9. ...a time when you were in good control of a situation.
10. ...a time when someone else really understood you.
11. ...a time when you really understood someone.
12. ...a recent time when you shared someone's world.
13. ...a recent time when someone shared your world.
14. ...a recent time when you really liked someone.
15. ...a recent time when someone was really fond of you.
16. ...a recent time when you felt in good communication with someone.
17. ...a recent time when you felt a strong sense of reality.
18. ...a recent time when you understood someone.
19. ...a recent time when someone really understood you.
20. ...a recent time when you were in good control of something.

Finally, do not ask about earlier incidents; one event per item is sufficient, and you can go through the list more than once if you need to. Usually that will not be required.

CASE HISTORIES AND TRANSCRIPTS

11

We devote a significant part of the training done during the four-day TIR workshop to watching and discussing videotaped sessions, and to having students both give and receive sessions in dyads. Although we realize that nothing can really adequately substitute for observing and participating in live sessions with supervision, this chapter is an attempt to provide the reader with something at least roughly analogous to that experience.

The first transcript is of an entire session of Basic TIR in an annotated form. We have included it here so that the reader might develop some feeling for the timing and emotional ebb and flow of a typical session, something it is impossible to do when one looks at such sessions piecemeal.

This viewer, a widow in her mid-sixties who lived with her daughter and son-in-law, had lost one of her two cats, a pet that she had dearly loved. It was an event that most would consider perhaps indeed upsetting but hardly traumatic—in the DSM-IV sense. Nonetheless, a number of her memories involved ugly incidents with the cat leading up to its death. Within a year after the death, these had become flashbacks which were occurring daily and had become extremely troubling to her. They were, in fact, her central presenting complaint. As well, since the death of the first, she had become obsessively concerned with the health of her other pet, a dog that displayed no symptoms at all.

The worst of the pictures haunting the viewer was of a specific incident. Because that incident was also the one that most strongly captured her interest in session, her facilitator—with her agreement, of course—chose to address it. As the item of concern was a specific incident rather than a theme, the facilitator used Basic TIR. (There did turn out to be an earlier incident, though, as is sometimes the case with Basic TIR. See Chapter 6.)

BASIC TIR—ALICE

Alice had had prior experience with therapy, including a number of hours aimed directly but unsuccessfully at resolving her presenting complaint. Whereas she felt that she had benefited significantly from her earlier counseling, she had come away from the more recent and unsuccessful sessions feeling, as she put it, "somewhat mauled". Thus, following the intake session and initial interview, her facilitator began her work in the second session by Unblocking (see Chapter 8) the subject of "the unsuccessful therapy"—the client's wording. After the facilitator devoted some time to explaining the procedure, the Unblocking itself took not quite 30 minutes to reach an end point. At the end of the session, facilitator and client agreed on a date and time for an extended session in which to do TIR.

The facilitator devoted the first minutes of the third session to explaining the TIR procedure, and to taking the viewer through a practice run on a nontraumatic incident. Then they took up the key incident, as follows:

Facilitator: When did it happen?
Alice: About three and a half years ago.
Facilitator: OK. How long does it last?

Note: We had not yet included Bisbey's "WHERE" question in the TIR protocol at the time of this session.

Alice: Well, it was a series of incidents with him, but this one
                incident in particular lasted, uh, a full day...a full day.
Facilitator: OK. I'd like you to go to the start of the incident and tell
                me when you've done so.

This is a less-than-textbook-perfect session, if only because the facilitator has varied the wording of the START instruction, above, in an effort, one supposes, to make the instruction more friendly. As you will see, she does more of the same elsewhere, and it is really neither necessary nor advisable, per our observations concerning the handling of communication in session. She gets away with it here, but might not have with another viewer.

Alice:	Yes.
Facilitator:	All right. What are you aware of?
Alice:	I'm aware of the sound of your pen...and a car horn...

An example follows of the use of Handling Originations, based on the facilitator's observation that the client has either forgotten or misunderstood the intent of the question, "What are you aware of?" The facilitator is not, of course, asking what the viewer is aware of in the room and time where the TIR session is taking place. Rather, she seeks the client's awareness of elements present in the "still photograph" that exists at—and will be used to "mark" for future reference—the start of the incident.

Facilitator:	OK, thanks. Now remember the "still photo" we talked about a few minutes ago—the one that contains whatever was present at the very beginning of the incident, just before the incident started?
Alice:	Yes....
Facilitator:	Good. Now I'm going to tell you to return to the moment that incident began—the time of the "photo"—and when you've done that, then I'll ask you what you're aware of, meaning "What do you see...or have an impression of...in the 'photograph' there at the start of the incident," OK?
Alice:	Oh, not...I'm...oh, yes, I thought you meant what was I aware of *here!* Got lost there for a second....
Facilitator:	All right. OK now?
Alice:	Yes, I got it.
Facilitator:	Good. Then let me have you go to the start of the incident and tell me when you've done so.

At this point the facilitator has returned the client to the procedure—albeit as noted above with a slight variation on the START instruction—and her use of Handling Originations is complete. The handling could perhaps have been a bit less cumbersome and lengthy and thus a bit more elegant, thereby drawing a bit less of the viewer's attention to the facilitator. Instead of reminding the viewer of the photo analogy, for instance, the facilitator might simply have acknowledged the viewer's answer to the (misunderstood) question, then repeated the instruction to go to the start of the incident, and then simply expanded the "aware of" question slightly, and gently, along the lines of "What are you aware of there...just at the start of the incident?" but though her handling was perhaps somewhat less than perfectly efficient, it was not wrong. She did:

1. understand *the viewer's confusion*
2. acknowledge *the viewer's answer*
3. resolve *the viewer's concern/problem*
4. return *the viewer to the next step of the procedure*

And as we stated earlier, that is as rote as one can make the exercise of Handling Originations.

Alice:	Yes.
Facilitator:	All right. What are you aware of?
Alice:	I'm aware of...uh...it was maybe two in the afternoon, and I was working in the garden...and it was a hot day...
Facilitator:	All right. Go through the incident to the end.
Alice:	*[19-second silent review]* Yes...OK....
Facilitator:	All right. Tell me what happened.
Alice:	I was on my hands and knees weeding in the yard, and I heard one of the animals...*howling*...Elsie...and it was a different...I dunno...it was just...awful, you know, just like a...screeching and, uh, I'd never heard that before. So I remember going in the door to the garage and she was there on the ground...uh...she looked like she was having an epileptic attack. And I remember screaming for my daughter, and she came running in from the kitchen. We really didn't know what to do, and...and...this attack went on...gosh...it seemed like...it seemed like a long time, but I think it was about...seven...eight minutes. *[This is all said in a ruminative, reflective tone.]* Yes. I want to say seven...17 minutes or something, but I...now that I'm looking at it, I think it was only seven or eight minutes, and, uh...and then she...just lay there, she just...she couldn't move, and, uh, we didn't know what to do, so we packed her off to the vet, and they couldn't find anything. Kept her in the hospital clinic overnight. She was fine in the morning as if...as if nothing had ever happened and, so they...they didn't know what it was, but she had another one. It was that afternoon. In the afternoon we brought her back

from the vet and he said, "There's nothing wrong"...She had another one of these attacks. So we took her back and, uh....

The viewer has completed a relatively matter-of-fact description of the incident and is starting to expand her view to include another, later incident. If permitted to continue, this would broaden the focus of the TIR excessively. Thus, the facilitator correctly takes her earliest opportunity and—with proper use of an acknowledgment in order to control (in this case, to stop) the communication—returns the viewer to the proper place in the "script".

Facilitator: OK. I wonder...could you go to the start of the incident and tell me when you're there.

Again, the wording change ("I wonder ... could you...?") was unnecessary and—although minor—a potential distraction to the viewer.

Alice: Uh, huh...I'm there.
Facilitator: Go through the incident to the end.

Facilitator forgets acknowledgment. While not necessarily very significant on a single occasion, the practice, if habitual—which, with this facilitator, it is not—is damaging.

Alice: *[13-second silent review]* Yes...
Facilitator: All right. Tell me what happened.
Alice: I could hear my cat...one of them...Elsie...and I thought I recognized it as her. I went running in the garage and she was writhing on the, uh...on the floor *[choked voice...grief]*. It was really ugly...to see....

Very significant change in affect. The facilitator simply (and quite correctly) continues.

Facilitator: OK. Go to the start of the incident and tell me when you've done so.
Alice: I'm having trouble hearing that, uh...howls? That's what I'm hearing....
Facilitator: All right. Go to the start of the incident and tell me when you've done so.

Alice:	Yes.
Facilitator:	All right. Go through the incident to the end.
Alice:	*[14-second silent review]* Yes...
Facilitator:	All right. Tell me what happened.
Alice:	On my knees there...and I heard...a howling. I was terrified. I didn't know what had happened, and when I ran in the garage, I could...I could see her just... convulsing.... And my daughter came out. Both of us were in a panic. We couldn't... Wanting to lean on one another and not really...nobody knew who to lean on. With all of my medical background, I, uh, knew what to do with people; I didn't know what to do with cats. And hear them scream. So we were both kind of...looking at one another and saying, "What do we *do?*" We had to go to an emergency because our vet...wasn't sure if our vet was in. We hadn't had to take them very much to the vet there. So we were both...now that I look at it, we're both kind of looking at one another to... "*You* take care of it! *You* do something!" Neither of us knows what to do at all. We just...were kinda locked into that panicking....I guess... that's what I remember....

Notice the viewer's brief excursion into the use of the present tense—neither a necessary nor sufficient condition for full resolution in a TIR session, but a positive indicator nonetheless, as noted elsewhere. Note also the phrase, "now that I look at it"—suggestive of the occurrence of at least a minor cognitive shift.

Facilitator:	All right. Go to the beginning of the incident and tell me when you've done so.
Alice:	The beginning seems easier...[indistinguishable]...
Facilitator:	All right. Go through the incident to the end.
Alice:	*[22-second silent review]* Yes...
Facilitator:	All right. Tell me what happened.
Alice:	My cat was howling...and my daughter and I were useless...just didn't know what to do. It was kinda like, uh...two people trying to...neither of us capable of holding the other up. We were just totally...out of our realm.
Facilitator:	All right. Go to the beginning of the incident and tell me when you've done so.

Here and elsewhere, the facilitator uses the word "beginning" instead of "start". It would not be a problem if she were being completely consistent, but she's not. She does get away with it, however, and most would with such a minor departure from the script. The devil, however, can definitely be in the details.

Alice:	Yes.
Facilitator:	OK. Go through the incident to the end.
Alice:	*[24-second silent review]* Yes...
Facilitator:	Tell me what happened.
Alice:	It gives a...screaming.... My daughter and I were just...we didn't really know how to touch her. We didn't know where she was hurt. There was no blood, there was nothing. She was just writhing...horribly...and I thought...I don't...I have no idea. I keep seeing it. My daughter looked in her mouth. She thought maybe she...Elsie...had gotten a bone or something, and, uh, there was nothing in her mouth and, uh, we just didn't know what to *do*, and so...she finally stopped. It seemed like forever, but she finally stopped this convulsion. I think my daughter said, "We have to take her to the vet"...and suddenly we're in the car, and going to the vet.... That's all....
Facilitator:	Go to the beginning of the incident and tell me when you have done so.

Another omitted acknowledgment....

Alice:	It's getting harder to go to the beginning.
Facilitator:	OK. Let me know if that changes. And I'll repeat the question...or the instruction.

This is a good, smooth handling by the facilitator of an unexpected communication by the viewer.

Alice:	OK.
Facilitator:	Good. Go to the start of the incident and tell me when you have done so.

Note again the inconsistency, between "start" and "beginning".

Alice:	OK.

Facilitator:	All right. Go through the incident to the end.
Alice:	*[21-second silent review]* Yes...
Facilitator:	All right. Tell me what happened.
Alice:	*[There is a sudden explosion of grief from the viewer, lasting two minutes and ten seconds...sobbing...choked words. Dramatically altered affect ... not atypical of TIR.]* I look down...I'm sorry.... *[sobbing...continues sobbing, blows nose, sobs subsiding; viewer gives a brief mumbled synopsis of incident]*
Facilitator:	All right. Go to the start of the incident and tell me when you've done so.

No expression of sympathy whatsoever from the facilitator; just a good, quiet acknowledgment, followed by the next instruction. Absolutely correct, procedurally, and not at all disconcerting to the viewer, whose attention is (and remains) on the incident where it needs to be, and not on the facilitator.

Alice:	Yes.
Facilitator:	Thank you. Go through the incident to the end.
Alice:	*[20-second silent review]* Yes...
Facilitator:	OK. Tell me what happened.
Alice:	When I saw my cat, when I ...her squealing...it was so *terrifying*...we didn't really know how to help her....It was scary...pretty scary to have those feelings...of being totally powerless.

No more tears; viewer not happy or sounding especially relieved, but calmer.

Facilitator:	All right. Go to the start of the incident and tell me when you have done so.
Alice:	Yes....
Facilitator:	OK. Go through the incident to the end.
Alice:	*[21-second silent review]* Can't seem to go through the incident...I seem to be...at the end of it...you know. Something's changed. More at the end of it...about knowing what to do and, uh, moving out of panic and fear? I think it's...

Viewer's tone of voice sounds relatively unchanged from her previous iteration, yet her words suggest that a significant change may be occurring. This dissonance causes the facilitator to wonder whether she should continue to run the incident or to inquire after an earlier starting point or incident. So she asks:

Facilitator:	Does the incident seem lighter? or heavier?
Alice:	It seems like it's shifted. I'm not stuck in that...*howling?* *[the word said in a questioning tone...wondering]* That's kind of lighter, but...fear is still pretty heavy.

Facilitator takes that ambiguous answer as the equivalent of "I don't know" from the viewer, and thus asks after an earlier start:

Facilitator:	All right. Does this incident actually have an earlier starting point?
Alice:	*[six-second pause, "looking"]* No.
Facilitator:	All right. Is there an earlier, similar incident?
Alice:	*[ten-second pause]* Yeah...maybe so, actually. I think so....
Facilitator:	OK. When did it happen?
Alice:	It was just...when I was just a little kid. I was...five...five...around sixty years ago....
Facilitator:	OK. How long does it last?
Alice:	A couple of years...I guess. It goes...the initial telling lasts a couple of minutes, but, uh, the effect lasts a long time.
Facilitator:	OK. So the actual incident itself lasts...?

Efficient, minimalist handling by the facilitator here of an ambiguous answer (hence, an origination) by the viewer.

Alice:	Maybe...three minutes.
Facilitator:	OK. Go to the start of the incident and tell me when you have done so.
Alice:	OK.
Facilitator:	*[missing acknowledgment]* What are you aware of?
Alice:	I'm aware of hearing my older sister over next to me, saying that, uh, Sparky, our dog, is missing, and I know I'm feeling...panic.
Facilitator:	*[missing acknowledgment]* Go through the incident to the end.
Alice:	*[19-second silent review]* Yes.
Facilitator:	*[missing acknowledgment]* Tell me what happened.

Alice:	We have this...mutt...a German Shepherd mix. Sparky. She was a stray. We fed her, and had her for a few years, and, uh, everybody thought she was my sister's dog, but I was really attached to her and so hearing that she was missing, that was really difficult for me. *[Quiet tears.]* My sister... my sister wasn't *doing* anything...and it was supposed to be her dog. She wasn't doing anything. She wasn't...I don't remember if *she* was sad or anything. I just felt she wasn't *doing* anything. She wasn't...going out and *looking* for her...Sparky...and so I picked up my coat and I went out looking for her, high and low.
Facilitator:	OK. Go to the start of the incident and tell me when you've done so.
Alice:	Yes....
Facilitator:	*[missing acknowledgment]* Go through the incident to the end.
Alice:	*[25-second silent review]* Yes.
Facilitator:	All right. Tell me what happened.
Alice:	I hear my sister saying that my dog is missing...I'm feeling really scared *[sniffs]* ...and sad. My sister doesn't make any moves...to go and *do* anything. Inside of me, there's all of this...this *fear*...and wondering what *happened*, and...I just...don't see my sister...*[long, reflective pause; beginning of a smile]* it's that she wasn't taking care of my *fear!* *[laugh]* But she didn't *know* anything *about* it! How *could* she have? I didn't *tell* her!

As noted elsewhere, this sort of entirely spontaneous cognitive shift is a not-uncommon component of end points in all metapsychological procedures, certainly including TIR. This one is especially typical, involving as it does the viewer's recognition of her own responsibility for—and hence, by implication, her ability to control—the reaction that she had had at the time of the incident and which had appeared to her, ever since, to be an essential and immutable aspect of the experience and its aftermath. This is a good example of an inflow becoming a reflexive flow upon review.

Alice:	*[Laugh]* But somehow...anyway...she wasn't taking care of my fear, and she *should* have been aware that I loved that dog... and she just wasn't! And so I, uh...*[laughing]* I got

on my little coat, and out the door I went! That's what I did! *[laugh...big smile]*

At this point, the viewer's indicators have improved rapidly and very markedly. She's laughing and speaking in a joking tone, and the incident has lost its charge. Her tone makes it clear that she has realized that her sister was not really at fault as she had thought.

A more experienced facilitator than this one, having seen here all the elements of an end point—she has moved into the present and is extroverted, with insight and very good indicators—would have ended the procedure at this point, or else simply remained silent briefly to see if there might be anything else the viewer wished to say. Less elegantly but acceptably, she might have asked the viewer—after acknowledging the viewer's conclusion, of course—if she felt that that would be a good point at which to end the session.

In this instance, however, the inexperienced facilitator either acted on a misplaced belief (and evaluation) that the viewer's indicators weren't "good enough" or, more likely, as a result of her inexperience, simply failed to notice the conjunction of all the elements of an end point, and thus continued as if nothing had changed.

| Facilitator: | Go to the start of the incident and tell me when you've done so. |
| Alice: | OK.... |

This "OK" is said with some hesitancy, as if perhaps the viewer were puzzled by the instruction. Not surprising. She is being run past a good end point. Again, if the facilitator had been more experienced, she would have noticed the hesitancy in the viewer's response, and queried it, per the section in Chapter 4 on Handling Originations. That doesn't happen here. Rather, she simply continues the TIR, instructing the viewer to review the incident.

| Facilitator: | Go through the incident to the end. |
| Alice: | *[One-minute and 47-second silent review]* Yes . . . . |

During the silence, an uncharacteristically long review for this particular viewer, the facilitator begins to introvert herself, wondering if she's done something wrong... which, of course, she has. The immediate and predictable result of this small bout of self-criticism is that the attention she has been devoting to the session and the viewer flags, and she makes another and—to the viewer—more obvious mistake: she "loses her place", and inadvertently repeats an instruction that this viewer has already carried out.

Facilitator: All right. Go through the incident to the end.
Alice: Yes.

Viewer gives this response almost instantaneously, and in a faintly impatient tone. It is clear that if she had been more assertive, she would have said something along the lines of, "I already did that!" The facilitator's error has caused the viewer's earlier delight in her realization to be replaced with irritation at the facilitator's failure to simply acknowledge her. It is really a reverse of the example we gave in Chapter 4 in which the wife asks what time it is, her husband responds with a negative concern, and the wife just repeats her question without acknowledging the concern in any way. In the present instance, it is as if the husband/viewer has said something like, "Hey, guess what? My sister's company got the funding!" and the wife/facilitator has responded with, "Let me ask you again: what time is it?" The viewer's attention has been stripped from the incident and placed squarely on the facilitator.

Facilitator: Tell me what happened.

This instruction is followed by another long silence, during which the facilitator notes the less-than-very-good indicators in the viewer and decides—correctly, and only somewhat belatedly—that something has gone awry and that an attempt to find out what it might have been and how to fix it is in order. Thus, she interrupts the silence with what, under the circumstances, is a good question:

Facilitator: Let me ask you another question: has anything occurred
                 in the past few minutes?
Alice: Well...yeah, maybe.
Facilitator: All right, tell me about it....
Alice: I dunno... I...just thinking about the dog.... *[pause]*
Facilitator: Uh-huh....
Alice: I started feeling pretty good about something I've felt bad
                 about for a long time...
Facilitator: Tell me what happened?
Alice: Well, when I was thinking about hearing that our dog was
                 missing, and about my sister not doing anything, I, uh...

[long, reflective pause] I got this clear picture *[laugh]* of my getting up and *doing* something! I don't know how useful it was...I didn't find Sparky. But...I got up and *did* something! And it related to...I didn't see much of a connection between Elsie's convulsions and that last silly incident when it popped up...when you asked about similar...but I think it was the blaming myself and my daughter for *not* doing anything. I mean...when we really *did* do something. The *right* thing *[laugh]* ...the *only* thing we could have done. We took her to the vet....

The viewer has extroverted again, is expanding on her realization, and her good indicators have returned; the end point has been "recovered".

Alice: It's like I've been feeling...*guilty?* yeah, guilty!...for all this time...which feels stupid now. I don't *have* to anymore! *[big smile]*

Facilitator: Seem like a good place for us to end the session?

Alice: *[Somewhat surprised...then happy]* Oh...? Actually, yes...yes! That's great.

Facilitator: OK, that's all on that.

Alice: *[Silent...growing smile...then]* Thanks. That's...really nice.

At this point, the facilitator declared the session finished.

BASIC TIR—MARY

Mary is a woman in her early fifties. The traumatic event that she addressed with TIR occurred while she was in a cabin on a wilderness hiking trip in Colorado with her husband and friends who owned a large Doberman mix named Rebel. One morning, without warning, Rebel attacked and savaged her arm and wrist terribly before the others were able to drag him away from her. Her husband had a satellite-linked phone and she was taken to a hospital by helicopter. The incident took place seven years prior to her experience with TIR and traumatized her severely, both physically and emotionally. It resulted in wounds which required surgery at the time and on three subsequent occasions, and years of physical therapy to restore the full use of her right hand. It also led to full-blown PTSD.

Over the years following the mauling, Mary acquired virtually the entire panoply of DSM-IV PTSD symptoms, including nightmares and flashbacks. Even after her wounds had healed sufficiently to permit her to hold a steering wheel and drive a car, she remained controlled by her fears and gave up driving lest she encounter a dog—even one that she "knew to be friendly and gentle". Walking alone beyond the confines of her house became out of the question. Her marriage came under severe strain, and many of her friends drifted away from her. On numerous occasions, triggers such as the sound of a gate latch rattling "like a dog's chain" or the sight of a dog or anything that even vaguely resembled a dog—such as a dog's picture in a magazine, the appearance of one in a movie she was attending, the strap of a woman's handbag that resembled a leash, or even a mop of curly hair on a child's head—caused her literally to run, terrified and screaming, from the trigger. On one occasion, panicked and hysterical at the sight of a blind man with a guide dog, she clambered whimpering over the people sitting in the rows of seats behind her at a concert.

Mary saw a psychologist weekly for the next six years without significant change. He referred her to a specialist in behavior therapy, who referred her, in turn, to a specialist in PTSD ("He saw me for a long time and then told me he couldn't help me; I said 'good-by'."), to an M.D. for medications ("He put me on anti-depressants and they had too many side effects"), and to yet another who was more familiar with PTSD and whom Mary saw for ten visits ("But I thought he was even less helpful. It didn't work at all.") The behaviorist then sent her to a therapist trained in a radically "different" short-term therapy—Eye Movement Desensitization and Reprocessing (EMDR). She had three sessions with that specialist, to no avail. Her symptoms persisted and were worsening. Desperate, Mary agreed to spend two weeks in a hospital for treatment and observation. Shortly before she was to go in, however, her therapist encountered a description of TIR in a literature search and described it in turn to Mary as "...something that might be worth a try". Mary agreed. He located a TIR-trained facilitator, and Mary went to see him. During her initial interview, Mary gave her history, summarizing the changes that the trauma had wrought in her life with the statement: "I used to feel free; now I don't."

She was taking Valium (.5 mg/night for sleep), Xanax (25mg 5X/day), and other medications on which she agreed to cut back before attempting TIR. She presented with pressured speech and agitated depression. She had a lot of attention on the continuing failure of therapy to help her, describing at length a number of problems and misgivings she had had concerning the therapy she had been through since the event: "The sessions were over so fast that it was difficult to trust", "My agenda didn't seem to be as important as the therapists' agenda", "By the time I started a session, it was time to stop", "The doctor said I was 'doing better on medication' when I knew I wasn't", "I've felt diminished by most of them [her therapists] because they've always told me what's wrong with me".

Mary's prior experience with other interventions had been extensive and largely negative. As we noted earlier, such past failures often tend to color a client's perceptions and expectations of current therapy. Knowing this, the facilitator elected, before attempting TIR, to give Mary a session devoted to Unblocking on the subject of prior efforts to help her. The Unblocking session went very well and reached a good end point. The facilitator then scheduled an open-ended session with Mary in which to address the core incident with Basic TIR. The following is a transcript of one of the passes through the incident of the attack; it is representative of many of the run-throughs:

> Facilitator: Go to the start of the incident and tell me when you have done so.
>
> Mary: OK, I'm there....

Since this is not the first pass through the incident, the facilitator does not ask Mary what she is aware of at this point.

> Facilitator: All right. Go through the incident to the end.
>
> Mary: *[three-minute and seven-second silent review]* OK.

Note that the time required for this step of silent viewing varies greatly from viewer to viewer and even within a single session with the same viewer.

> Facilitator: Good. Tell me what happened.
>
> Mary: I'm sitting on a log bench outside the cabin....It's a warm day, and Sam and the Morrises have gone for a walk down near the stream. I'm thirsty, and...actually, the pump wasn't around the left side of the cabin, come to think of it, it was on the right...I'm going towards it....

In earlier passes, Mary has said she was going to the left. The change in the story line—trivial in this instance, but sometimes very major—is typical of TIR. Do such altered perceptions represent closer approximations of some absolute truth?

To anyone operating under the Rules of Facilitation, it doesn't matter. Should the changed perception be regarded as an "inconsistency" and disputed or even simply queried by the facilitator? Never.

> Mary: ...yeah...I walk around the corner of the cabin towards the pump...

The viewer's voice, fairly calm and matter-of-fact to this point, now breaks, her words becoming rushed, her speech pressured.

> Mary: ...and then there's this flash of black and I felt these teeth...and he grabbed me...before I knew it, it was Rebel [the dog]...

Mary's voice has rapidly become a high, keening wail that quickly becomes a sort of nonstop, choked and muffled screaming.

> Mary: ...and he grabbed me but I looked down really far...it was behind...and I saw him, he was in like...hanging from my arm...and I saw...and he was grabbing me...and he was going back and forth with his head...and he was growling...and he was biting me...and I didn't know what to do...I didn't know what to do...I'm holding onto the pump...and I'm pulling...and I'm pulling...

Now Mary is completely "in" the incident. Her words are coming out in a torrent, and she is employing the present tense exclusively. Close to hyperventilation, she utters single words and short phrases with each rapid exhalation in the high, frantic voice described above.

> Mary: ...I'm pulling the pump with all my strength...I'm holding onto the pump with all my strength...I'm pulling...and I'm holding and...and he's pulling me...and he's shaking me...and he's shaking me up...and I'm so scared...oh...oh...oh...he has my arm...and he's pulling my arm...and he's pulling my arm...and there he's eating me...he's eating me up and I can't get away...I can't get away...I don't want to fall down...I'm trying not to...he's gonna grab my arm...he's gonna grab my wrist...and he's shaking my...his head back and forth...

At this point, still in a frantic rush, Mary begins to speak in whispered phrases.

Mary: …oh not that…it was so loud…it was so loud…it was so loud…he was…he's growling…growling…he was biting…he was pulling…he's pulling…he's pulling…he's pulling…he's pulling me…he's pulling me…he's pulling it…and I…nobody was coming, I…oh-hhh…nobody's coming, nobody's coming…no…he wasn't coming…he wasn't coming … no … no … no…no … no … nobody's coming … oh … oh … oh … oh …

Mary is hyperventilating; in and out of present tense.

Mary: he's pulling…pulling…really…oh…no…he's pulling…now he's stopping…I thought I thought I was gonna get away…just for a second…and it wasn't working…and he went ahead…and he grabbed me again…on the wrist…and I looked at the blood all over my shirt…no…it can't be me…and it was me…and it was me, and I was so…oh, I was screaming, screaming at what was happening…no!… no!…no!…no!…I heard some voices in the background…towards the stream…they weren't coming. Why were they not coming?…Why were they not coming? No, come on…come on, come and get me…Why me? Why me? No, it hurts so bad. I'm so scared…I'm being eaten alive…No! No! No! No! No! No! No! No!

The "No's gradually become almost a scream. Then Mary gradually slows down, as if exhausted at the end of a race.

Mary: And it hurts! Rebel!…Rebel!…Rebel!…Come and get me! Hurry up…hurry up… hurry up…hurry up…hurry up…no…no…no…no…no…no…well, hurry up…OK…all right…I didn't feel anything…they took him off me…oh…oh…I tell Sam…Sam, it hurts so bad… Sam, help me…oh…oh…oh…and he walked me over to the bench…oh…and he held my…my hand…by the bench…and he took off my shirt…and it was all blood…there was so much blood…oh…oh…oh…and they gave me some medicine...oh...couldn't believe it happened...where have you been?...oh, it hurts so bad....oh...oh...oh... *[long pause]* Then it's sort of...numb....I was in shock....Peter called civilization and got a Medivac for me....

Then Mary sighs and indicates that she is through with that pass; the facilitator acknowledges, and returns her to the beginning of the incident for the next pass. There are elements in the story that conflict—"I didn't feel anything" and "it hurts so bad", for example—a fact that is, again, quite irrelevant in the context of TIR.

Following a total of 22 iterations of this event, each one tending to require less time than the ones before (as is typical in TIR), Mary spotted and described an earlier, related incident which went to a full end point in 11 passes. Some days after the TIR, Mary called her facilitator and told him: "I have an enormous smile on my face, and I think it's going to stay there." During the months since then, she has been completely comfortable walking and driving by herself. She states that she feels "free" again, for the first time in seven years. She has been off medications entirely since the first session, and has had no difficulty when exposed to things that have always acted as triggers in the past, frequently not even noting their presence until her husband points one out "and both of us laugh about it": she can touch and hold dogs, a fact she finds utterly astonishing, and has even been able—to her enormous delight—to deliberately put her hand inside the mouth of a dog she knew to be gentle. She speaks with much less pressured speech, and has not had any more nightmares or flashbacks at all. And she has bought a dog of her own.

BASIC TIR—JOHN

John is a tall, muscular Vietnam vet in his early forties [13]. In an initial interview, it was found that he had increasing difficulty after returning from more than a year of intense combat experience in the Special Forces. He had severe, persistent nightmares and anxiety attacks in which he continually relived battle scenes. At the time of the interview, John had just completed many months of therapy at a government-sponsored center for the treatment of PTSD, but his symptoms remained unabated or worsened.

When he was asked to find a traumatic incident, John did so without hesitation. In fact, he was already "in" a specific incident that had haunted him for more than 20 years. His facilitator directed him through this first incident 17 times. Each time, John described it in detail, though different details kept appearing. Initially, John ran the incident calmly and dispassionately. After several passes, however, he was manifesting an enormous amount of grief and terror as he recounted the events it contained. With further repetition, the intensity of negative emotion gradually diminished, until after 13 or 14 run-throughs he was again able to recount the incident quite calmly. The facilitator made no comment whatsoever about what John was saying, but simply acknowledged him and continued to direct him through the incident. At the end of 50 minutes, John brightened up and laughed, and the session ended. He was tired but "feeling good".

Significantly, he noted the fact that although this incident had come up repeatedly in his previous therapy, he had never before been given the opportunity to go through it even *once* without being interrupted by questions, interpretations, evaluations, and invalidations.

In four subsequent sessions, John handled four more incidents, with an average of 14 repetitions per incident and 58 minutes per session. At that point, though his life was far from perfect, John was (and would remain) completely free of the nightmares, anxiety attacks, and flashbacks that he had suffered for many years. He described himself as "happy to be alive" and said he no longer felt fixed in the identity of a Vietnam veteran. "I don't have to keep *being* a Vietnam vet. I can *stop!*", as he put it. During his sessions, he had many insights and realizations, all completely self-generated.

John's incidents were all "self-contained", and each surrendered fairly easily to straightforward Basic TIR with only a single incident needing to be addressed. As mentioned earlier, however, incidents that seem likely to be self-contained—to have involved sufficient obvious, known trauma and emotional charge to constitute their own root, so to speak—will sometimes prove nonetheless to depend from other, earlier incidents.

THE UNEXPECTED ROOT

As can be seen from the cases of Mary and Alice, it is a mistake to assume that the earliest traumatic event in a sequence of related incidents—the root incident—will always and inevitably be "worse" than any later ones depending from it, in any objectively measurable sense. In the case of Mary's mauling, for example, the root incident—the one that eventually went to a full end point—involved no major physical trauma whatsoever. Rather, it involved "only" a trivial injury received as a child. Yet the later and seemingly vastly more severe trauma of having been attacked and mauled by the dog did not resolve until the viewer had addressed and handled the charge from the earlier incident.

Perhaps the single most dramatic instance that either of us has ever encountered of the incongruity between a seemingly "light" but nonetheless root incident and a horrific secondary incident connected to it, transpired during a session in which neither the facilitator nor the viewer spoke a word of the other's language. The entire session took place with a translator—herself observing the Rules of Facilitation—making communication possible between the facilitator and the viewer. It represents part of a growing body of evidence, albeit anecdotal, suggesting that the effectiveness of TIR may be culture-blind.

BASIC TIR—GABRIELLE

Gabrielle is Egyptian, and lived with her husband in a wealthy suburb of Cairo. One night when their only child, Marionette, 23 years old, had come for a visit, three armed men, all apparently on drugs, broke into the house. The family was alone having dinner. The men demanded money, and when Gabrielle's husband did not move quickly enough to suit them, one of them stabbed him repeatedly, killing him in front of his wife and daughter. Gabrielle screamed; Marionette fainted. Another of the men, laughing, leaned over and shot her in the head as she lay on the floor at her mother's feet, killing her instantly. Gabrielle begged the men to kill her, too. Cursing and laughing, they gagged her, tied her to a heavy banister, and fled the house, taking with them a small television set and some pieces of silverware.

Following this horrendous event, Gabrielle developed full-fledged PTSD. She saw numerous therapists during the ensuing year, none of whom were able to help her. Among the symptoms she acquired were heavy depression, listlessness, flashbacks, and nightmares.

Two years after the incident, she was "finally able to feel safe with a man for the first time since it happened"; she fell in love and was able to talk to her new companion easily, but her symptoms persisted, and she found that despite wishing to, she was unable to consummate the new relationship.

The session in question came about as it did because Gabrielle's closest friend had gone to Greece on vacation with her husband. There the couple had met, enjoyed, and spent several days in the company of a young American lay counselor and her husband, an architect. The counselor had recently been trained in TIR and had been making extensive and successful use of it in her work. During conversation over dinner one evening, she happened to mention TIR and her enthusiasm for the tool, thus inadvertently initiating a discussion about Gabrielle. As it happened, the American couple had already planned a brief trip to Cairo, during which, with Gabrielle's agreement, the therapist arranged for a single open-ended TIR session to take place on the only day that the counselor had available.

Gabrielle had led a comfortable and relatively uneventful life prior to the night of the incident, had never used drugs or alcohol, was not taking any medicines that would interfere with her ability to run TIR, and was willing to attempt something "different from what the other therapists did" on the recommendation of her friend. In short, she seemed to be a good candidate for TIR. The counselor made no promises, but felt hopeful that even a single session would help, and Gabrielle's friend was able to communicate that hopefulness to her. The friend had agreed to act as translator after the therapist explained the procedure, the Rules of Facilitation, and what would be required of her in that role. She explained, for instance, that the vocal expressions of sympathy that the friend would normally be inclined to offer Gabrielle during the session would be very counterproductive in the work they'd be doing, and that it would be important for her to pass on just the simple acknowledgments that the therapist would be giving as facilitator.

The session of Basic TIR lasted approximately 2½ hours, and there was not anything unusual about the way it began, nor with how it progressed for the first 1 to 1½ hours. For the first few passes, Gabrielle told the story of the incident in a monotone voice with flat affect. She then contacted the suppressed emotional charge in the incident and proceeded through a number of iterations of the incident, alternating between anguished grief and anger. During the next 15 to 20 iterations of the incident, about 1½ hours into the session, the intensity of her affect tapered off into the appearance of "a sort of listless, apathetic resignation". Once she reached this plateau, Gabrielle remained there for pass after pass, with no further significant changes in affect, no major changes in the content of the narrative ... and no end point.

Recall that the protocol governing the use of Basic TIR dictates that when the facilitator observes such a "flat" pattern appearing *after* a number of iterations containing change, she should seek to discover, first, an earlier starting point and then, if there is none, an earlier incident, similar in some way to the one being run. In this instance, the therapist failed to do that, for the simple reason that she was absolutely *certain* that nothing "worse" than what she was hearing could possibly have happened to Gabrielle earlier in her life. Instead, she simply plowed ahead far longer than she had to, or should have, going over and over the incident involving the murder of the family long after procedural protocol would have had her ask for an earlier beginning or incident, no matter *what* she thought she "knew".

Finally, sure that nothing would come of it but beginning to feel somewhat desperate about where the session was (or, rather, was *not*) going, she did ask for earlier material. To her amazement, Gabrielle provided it—in the form of a seemingly trivial incident that had occurred when she was only six or seven years old, walking with her father and mother on a crowded city street in London where she and her mother had accompanied her father on a business trip. A man had run by them on the sidewalk, grabbing her mother's purse as he passed and tearing it away from her. Her father shouted and ran off in pursuit of the mugger, chasing him around a corner and out of sight. A short time later, he returned to Gabrielle and her mother, having been unsuccessful in his effort to run down the thief.

That was the entirety of the incident. Gabrielle's mother had been lightly bumped but was otherwise uninjured, and the man had touched neither Gabrielle nor her father. Yet this relatively innocuous event contained very significant emotional charge for Gabrielle. The later and seemingly much more horrendous incident in her adult life had triggered it, and that charge was sufficient to have held the later incident in place until Gabrielle contacted and resolved the earlier one.

Sometimes the facilitator never discovers exactly why such events contain as much charge as they do. The viewer simply reviews the earlier material one or more times and then reaches an end point without happening to provide the details to the facilitator that would allow the latter a full understanding of why the incident had such an effect. And the person-centered context essential to TIR forbids the sort of query after the fact that the facilitator might otherwise be inclined to make. In this case, though, Gabrielle did happen to explain: during the long few minutes that her father had been out of sight, Gabrielle had become convinced that he had been killed by the man he was chasing and would never return. However short-lived, that belief, of course, contained enormous charge—suppressed over the years, probably at least in part by her father's subsequent pooh-poohing of her terror.

THEMATIC TIR—DEAN

Dean was on patrol in Vietnam, momentarily alone and completely exposed in the open, when he came under sudden, heavy fire from an enemy ambush site [13]. He was wounded in the episode, and although other members of his patrol were under cover nearby and able to witness his situation, no one came to his immediate aid. The incident contained a number of themes and potential triggers/restimulators, including:

- Open spaces
- Panic
- (The feeling or fear of) being abandoned
- Rage
- Surprise and shock
- Loud noises (gunfire)

During an initial interview before his first session of TIR, Dean mentioned and briefly described this incident. He wept as he did so, and had difficulty saying the word "ambush", choking as he spoke it.

Some months after returning home from Vietnam, Dean was playing golf with his parents on the Fourth of July. As they approached the golf green, someone set off a firecracker in the distance. Dean suddenly found himself sprawled in a sand bunker in a state of hypervigilance, holding his golf club to his shoulder like a rifle. As he began to recover his composure, he saw his parents looking away from him ("abandoning" him), in an effort to ignore his bizarre reactions. This incident contained themes in common with the earlier one, as well as at least one new potential trigger and a new theme:

- Open spaces
- Loud noises
- Abandonment
- Surprise and shock
- *The game of golf* (new potential trigger)
- *Embarrassment* (new theme)

In the course of the same initial interview, Dean mentioned in passing that "golf is a stupid game", and that he "wouldn't be caught dead playing it". He also described the "excruciatingly painful embarrassment" he experienced in manifesting a "startle reaction" in public.

A few years later, Dean was walking along an unfamiliar city street. It was a normal business day, and his thoughts were elsewhere. As he turned a corner, a vagrant accosted him unexpectedly, demanding money in a threatening manner. Themes and triggers present in the incident included:

- Open spaces
- Fear
- Rage
- Surprise and shock
- *City streets* (new potential trigger)

By the time of his initial interview, Dean had come to generalize the threat in this incident and carry it over to all of his life. He stated that he was "forever grateful" that he had become an expert in martial arts, because "you never know when you'll get jumped".

Some years later, Dean experienced the disintegration of a close relationship. His partner told him that she intended to break off their relationship, that her plans were already implemented, and that she was leaving him that day, forever. The themes and triggers present in this incident included:

- Abandonment
- Rage
- Surprise and shock
- *A close relationship* (new potential trigger)

Dean's preliminary interview included statements by him: "It never pays to allow someone to become too close to you", and, "I'm a loner, and I'm capable of taking care of myself with no help from pseudo-friends, thank you!"

In Dean's case, a number of themes, each debilitating to a greater or lesser degree, were all linked to the same sequence of traumatic incidents, leading back to what turned out to be a root in the ambush he had experienced in Vietnam.

In a TIR session, pursuing one of the themes on which his attention had become riveted, Dean reviewed each of the incidents described, eventually reaching and running the root—the ambush. At that point, he experienced an insight concerning the similarities (themes) contained in the other incidents, and with an abruptness that is common in TIR, they ceased to trouble him. Since that session (both observably and—of far greater significance—in his own estimation), Dean has been able to discard his negative attitudes about golf and his fear of the dangers of city streets. He has come to regard his reflexes ("startle reaction") as a potential asset—something that no longer embarrasses him in the slightest, but of which, to the contrary, he is proud. He no longer fears emotional commitment—and he can comfortably recall the ambush experience, talk about it openly and candidly, and, in his words, "put it aside as one does the morning paper".

BASIC AND THEMATIC TIR—SEAN

Sean is yet another Vietnam combat veteran, a marine who presented with classic PTSD manifestations, most of which he had had for more than 20 years, and none of which had abated significantly during seven months of treatment he had recently received in an inpatient setting [13].

Before he began viewing, when his facilitator asked him what he hoped to gain from it, he said, "to be able to experience a single hour of uninterrupted happiness"—something that he said he had not experienced since prior to having gone to Vietnam in 1967 at the age of 18. Within 25 hours of working on specific incidents, Sean had attained this goal and in fact, with the exception of the physical "startle reaction", had seemingly eradicated all manifestations of PTSD.

At this point, the facilitator began addressing themes, pursuing each theme through earlier similar incidents to an end point. This continued for an additional five hours. Since then, the themes that Sean addressed with TIR have ceased to trouble him.

EPILOGUE

There is precious little research involving TIR. The present authors have unpublished informal case studies some of which have been detailed throughout this text. Such research is defined by Moon & Trepper [26, p. 393] as "clinical action research that is undertaken by clinicians who wish to…disseminate their clinical innovations to a wider audience through publication." By definition, this research is not quantitative and cannot meet strict positivistic assumptions for hypothesis testing. However, informal case studies are extremely flexible and allow for hypothesis generation, which is part of the sum and substance of this text. Therefore, these case studies are presented as descriptive and discovery oriented.

Further, the present authors utilized (in part) a research strategy based on the paradigm known as research and development (R&D) in industry. This strategy was particularly applicable in the early work of developing the TIR techniques—and continues to this day as we develop newer TIR-type interventions. Bischoff et al. [5] proposes that R&D techniques can be notably useful as they allow: (a) for ideas to be more quickly developed and adapted as specific modifications take place; (b) for the discarding of interventions that do not meet criteria; and (c) the researchers to identify the strengths and weaknesses of an intervention. The recursive sequences of R&D research include: designing the intervention, replicating the intervention, improving the intervention, replicating the improvements, modifying more if necessary, replicating the modifications, and deriving the final technique. One of the ideas proposed by Bischoff et al. [5] is that R&D research attempts to bridge a gap between interventions and therapy-seeking behavior by precisely estimating the needs of clients and attempting to meet those needs—again a goal of TIR.

Presently there is no outcome research in refereed journals pertaining to TIR efficacy. However there is doctoral research, a quantitative study in progress, and other pending work.

In her doctoral dissertation, Bisbey [4] utilized 57 participants diagnosed with PTSD in three separate conditions. The first was a treatment paradigm called direct therapeutic exposure (DTE) which is a pure exposure treatment. The second was TIR, an exposure treatment that explores cognitive content. The third was a control group. The conditions were short-term with 20 hours of treatment over five weeks. The outcome indicated both the DTE and TIR treatment paradigms showed significant improvement over the controls with the TIR group showing significantly more improvement than the DTE group. Bisbey [4] suggests the potential of examining cognitive content as being more effective than pure exposure treatments.

Those subjects who received TIR as a treatment assignment improved the most. These findings provided initial information on the effectiveness of TIR, and provided further information on the effectiveness of DTE, when working with crime victims who have PTSD. Of the subjects involved in this study, 82.2% were the victims of violent crime. The resulting improvement with short-term intensive therapy methods is very encouraging.

With the crime rate expanding, the importance of finding reliable and effective treatment methods for this population is clear. The more information practitioners and researchers have, the more likely they are to be able to reduce the effects of crime on the people who are victimized and, consequently, on society as a whole [3].

A three-year outcome-research endeavor is being undertaken by the Occupational Health department at London Transport, Ltd. Lori Beth Bisbey, Ph.D., C.T.S., C. Psychol., is the senior investigator. Dr. Bisbey's research [3] is a treatment outcome study comparing TIR to DTE and eye movement desensitization and reprocessing (EMDR) [27] with London Transport employees who have PTSD following a variety of traumatic events, the two most common having been assaults and train suicides (i.e., drivers who have experienced people throwing themselves under their trains). Bisbey intends to have more than 100 participants before it ends and there are four research clinicians (two men and two women) working with the three treatment paradigms.

All participants will receive up to 20 hours of treatment in sessions that are two hours in length, twice per week if possible. Presently, 48 participants have completed the treatments and there are six-month follow-up data on 10 of them, one-year follow-up data on 10, and two-year follow-up data on 3. Some of the participants are being screened out of the study using MMPI scales for fragility (i.e., not in good enough shape physically or emotionally to handle the requirements of the exposure-based treatment models). The acceptance criteria for participants in the study include:

1. diagnosis of PTSD from symptom checklist
2. diagnostic interview
3. no diagnosis of substance abuse or dependence that is active

Other measures being utilized in this research include the PENN Inventory, the Impact of Events Scale, and the MMPI-2 (basic, supplementary, and content scales).

To summarize this study to date (January, 1998), Bisbey [3] reports the London Transport staff in the treatment groups experienced a significant decrease in trauma-related symptoms as a result of treatment. All subjects qualified for a diagnosis of PTSD at the beginning of the study whereas at the end of the study many did not. Bisbey [3] suggests future research on these treatment methods could include an analysis of the principal components of the treatments in order to discover what components make the treatments successful. Research that examines the relationship between other types of psychopathology, symptomatology, and treatment outcome with TIR and DTE would also help answer some of the questions raised about treatment matching by the researchers in this study.

The importance of treatment outcome research in understanding and resolving PTSD cannot be stressed enough. The Bisbey research has raised interesting questions about theoretical issues in PTSD and further investigation could lead to: (a) more integrative theory; and (b) consequently more reliable and effective treatment methods.

Joyce Carbonell and Charles Figley of Florida State University began a study in 1993 of four major "power therapies", as they have come to be known, which include TIR, EMDR, Thought Field Therapy (TFT), and Visual-Kinesthetic Dissociation (VKD). According to an article in *The Family Therapy Networker*, written by Wylie [32], the study (not yet published as of January, 1998) was designed to evaluate these therapeutic models on actual clients.

The group of clients treated with TIR were similar to those treated by the other approaches. They were predominantly women, with a mean age of 41, and on the average, had more than a high school education. The problems presented by the clients varied greatly, but as with the overall sample (n = 51), the most frequent problem presented was a history of childhood abuse. Each client who came to treatment were treated by one of the three TIR therapists who participated in the study. Given the nature of TIR, the length of therapy varied greatly by client. On the average, clients were seen for a total of approximately four hours.

Although the intent was to ask each client for a Subjective Unit of Distress (SUD)* rating before and after treatment, much of this data is missing for TIR, as it was not part of the normal protocol. However, on an anecdotal level, clients reported considerable relief and improvement immediately after treatment. Post-testing after six months clearly indicates a decrease in the reporting of symptoms across several measures, the Brief Symptom Inventory (BSI) and the Impact of Events Scale (IES) and SUD.

Subject scores decreased on all three of the global measures on the BSI. The Intrusion and Avoidance scales of the IES also demonstrated a decrease with clients going from a high score to a medium score on the avoidance subscale. Although there was also a decrease on the Intrusion subscale from high to medium, it was not as large a change as was obtained on the avoidance scale. Once again, this is based on only a part of the sample (n = 5), as following the subjects across a six-month period proved difficult and the majority of the sample was not available for follow up.

We would like to invite and encourage research which can provide both quantitative and qualitative explorations of TIR and its use and efficacy with a wide variety of psychological problems.

Finally, it is our wish that the publication of this text will give new hope to those who work and live with PTSD. The product of a paradigm that both perceives and places great healing powers in the hands of those who would be healed, TIR is a tool capable of rapidly and profoundly improving those lives most desperately in need of transformation.

---

* A self-report scale from 1 to 10 where 1 represents the least distress felt and 10, the most.

REFERENCES

1. American Psychiatric Association (1994). *Diagnostic and statistical manual of mental disorders, fourth edition.* Washington, D. C.: American Psychiatric Association.

2. American Psychiatric Association (1980). *Diagnostic and statistical manual of mental disorders, third edition.* Washington, D. C.: American Psychiatric Association.

3. Bisbey, L. B. (1997). Personal communication via e-mail documents, computer filed as Bisbeys #1, Bisbeys #2, and Bisbeys #3.

4. Bisbey, L. B. (1995). *No longer a victim: A treatment outcome study of crime victims with posttraumatic stress disorder.* Doctoral Dissertation, California School of Professional Psychology, San Diego, January.

4a. Bisbey, L. B. (1993). *The Newsletter of the Institute for Research in Metapsychology,* Vol. VI, 1.

5. Bischoff, R. J.; McKeel, A. J.; Moon, S. M.; & Sprenkle, D. H. (1996). Systematically developing therapeutic techniques: Applications of research and development. In D. H. Sprenkle & S. M. Moon (Eds.), *Research methods in family therapy.* New York: The Guilford Press.

6. Campbell, D.; Draper, R; & Crutchley, E. (1991). The Milan systemic approach to family therapy. In A. S. Gurman & D. P. Kniskern (Eds.), *Handbook of family therapy,* Volume II. New York: Brunner/Mazel.

7. Corey, G.; Corey, M.; & Callanan, P. (1993). *Issues and ethics in the helping professions,* fourth edition. Pacific Grove, CA: Brooks/Cole.

8. Coughlin, W. (1995). *Traumatic incident reduction: Efficacy in reducing anxiety symptomology.* Doctoral Dissertation, Union Institute, Cincinnati, OH, May.

9. Das, Babba Ram (1971). *Be here now.* Crown Publishing.

10. Figley, C. R. (1985). From victim to survivor: Social responsibility in the wake of catastrophe. In C. R. Figley (Ed.), *Trauma and its wake.* New York: Brunner/Mazel.

11. Figley, C. R. (1983). Catastrophes: An overview of family reactions. In C. R. Figley & H. I. McCubbin (Eds.), *Stress and the family, Volume II, Coping with catastrophe.* New York: Brunner/Mazel.

12. Figley, C. R. (1995). *Compassion fatigue: Coping with secondary traumatic stress disorder in those who treat the traumatized.* New York: Brunner/Mazel.

13. French, G. & Gerbode, F. (1996). *The Traumatic Incident Reduction Workshop Manual.* Menlo Park, CA: IRM Press.

13a. Gerbode, F. A. (1988). Unblocking. *The Journal of Metapsychology,* Vol. I, p. 117. [Available from the Traumatic Incident Reduction Association (TIRA), 13 NW Barry Road, Suite 214, Kansas City, MO 64155-2728; phone: (816) 468-4945; fax: (816) 468-6656; e-mail: tira@tir.org; <http://www.tir.org>.]

13b. Gerbode, F. A. (1990). Repeating viewing instructions without variation. *The Journal of Metapsychology,* Vol. III, pp. 3–4. [Available from the Traumatic Incident Reduction Association (TIRA), 13 NW Barry Road, Suite 214, Kansas City, MO 64155-2728; phone: (816) 468-4945; fax: (816) 468-6656; e-mail: tira@tir.org; <http://www.tir.org>.]

14. Gerbode, F. A. (1995). *Beyond psychology: An introduction to metapsychology* (third edition). Menlo Park, CA: IRM Press.

15. Gerbode, F. A. & Moore, R. H. (1994). Beliefs and intentions in RET. *Journal of Rational-Emotive & Cognitive-Behavior Therapy,* 12, 27–45.

16. Gurman, A. S. & Kniskern, D. P. (1981). *Handbook of family therapy, Volume I.* New York: Brunner/Mazel.

17. Gurman, A. S. & Kniskern, D. P. (1991). *Handbook of family therapy, Volume II.* New York: Brunner/Mazel.

18. Harris, C. J. (1995). Sensory-based therapy for crisis counselors. In C. R. Figley (Ed.), *Compassion fatigue.* New York: Brunner/Mazel.

19. Harris, C. J. (1991). A family crisis intervention model for the treatment of post-traumatic stress reaction. *Journal of Traumatic Stress,* 4, 195–207.

20. Harris, C. J. & Linder, J. G. (1995). Communication and self care: Foundational issues. In B. H. Stamm (Ed.), *Secondary traumatic stress.* Lutherville, MD: Sidran.

21. Horowitz, M. J. (1976). *Stress response syndromes.* New York: Jason Aronson.

22. Janoff-Bulman, R. (1992). *Shattered assumptions.* New York: The Free Press.

23. Korzybski, A. (1948). *Science and sanity, third edition.* Lakeville, CT: The International Non-Aristotelian Library Publishing Company.

24. Lewis, B. A. & Pucelik, R. F. (1982). *Magic demystified.* Lake Oswego, OR: Metamorphous Press.

25. Moore, R. H. (1993). Traumatic incident reduction: A cognitive-emotive treatment of post-traumatic stress disorder. In W. Dryden & L. K. Hill (Eds.), *Innovations in rational-emotive therapy.* Newbury Park, CA: Sage Publications.

26. Moon, S. M. & Trepper, T.S. (1996). Case study research. In D. H. Sprenkle & Moon (Eds.), *Research methods in family therapy.* New York: The Guilford Press.

27. Shapiro, F. (1995). *Eye movement desensitization and reprocessing: Basic principles, protocols and procedures.* New York: The Guilford Press.

28. Stanton, M. D. (1981). Strategic approaches to family therapy. In A. S. Gurman & D. P. Kniskern (Eds.), *Handbook of family therapy, Volume I.* New York: Brunner/Mazel.

29. Trimble, M. R. (1985). Post-traumatic stress disorder: History of a concept. In C. R. Figley (Ed.), *Trauma and its wake*. New York: Brunner/Mazel.
30. van der Kolk, B. A. & McFarlane, A. C. (1996). The black hole of trauma. In B. van der Kolk, A. McFarlane, & L. Weisaeth (Eds.), *Traumatic stress*. New York: The Guilford Press.
31. van der Kolk, B. A.; Weisaeth, L.; & van der Hart, O. (1996). History of trauma in psychiatry. In B. van der Kolk, A. McFarlane, & L. Weisaeth (Eds.), *Traumatic stress*. New York: The Guilford Press.
32. Wylie, M. S. (1996). Researching PTSD: Going for the cure. *The Family Therapy Networker*. July/August.

INDEX

A

abuse, childhood, 164
acknowledgment, 29, 141. *see also*
    communication
    authority in statements, avoiding, 37–38
    communication cycle, 35–36. *see also*
        communication
    errors, 39
    evaluative, 35
    in example session, 47
    facilitator control, avoiding, 39, 40
    judgment, 37
    of origination, 56
    partial, 41–42, 48
    timing, 40
    tone, 42
    unencumbered, 35
    vocal inflection, 40
acute victimization, 2, 4, 7. *see also* chronic
    victimization
age, of viewer, 127–129
alcohol use by viewer, 126
antihistamine, 127
anti-psychotic medication, 127
anxiolytics, 127
assessment, 66, 67
    during basic traumatic incident reduction,
        101

definition, 68, 69
viewer interest, 69
assimilation, of traumatic event, 6
awareness, 33
awareness threshold, 67, 68

B

basic traumatic incident reduction, 15, 18.
    see also thematic traumatic
    incident reduction; traumatic
    incident reduction
    "Alice" case study, 136–147, 153
    annotated transcripts, 135–159
    AWARE step, 75–76, 87, 89
    choosing incident to run (INC), 72–73,
        87, 101
    clarifying length of incident with viewer,
        74, 87
    in conjunction with thematic traumatic
        incident reduction, 159
    earlier, similar incident (EI), 84–87
    earlier starting point questions (ES), 84,
        102
    emotional charge reduction, 79, 81–82
    end point, 82. *see also* end point
    facilitator instructions, 71
    facilitator shorthand, 72, 87
    flows, 101–102. *see also* flows

scale. *see* emotional scale
empowerment, 101, 115–117
end point, 14
  in children, 129
  conditions prohibiting, 24
  directing viewer's attention to, 44
  extroversion as sign of, 19, 20
  grief process, 70
  importance of concept, 16–17
  importance of reaching, 64
  indicators. *see* indicators
  phenomena, 18–19. *see also* indicators
  of symptoms and session, 53
  theme resolution, 39, 70
  unable to reach, 132–133
  unblocking, reaching during, 113
  viewer recognizes things brought on self, 100–101
euphoria, 127
exposure-based therapy, 22
extroversion (at end point), 19, 20
eye movement desensitization and reprocessing, 148, 162, 163

F

facilitator, 11. *see also* therapist's role in traumatic incident reduction
  poorly trained, 130–131
  /therapist distinction, 117, 120–122. *see also* therapist's role in traumatic incident reduction
false memories, 85
family therapy, 120, 121
Figley, Charles, 163
flashback, 32
flinching, 32
flooding, 14
flows. *see also* causation
  in basic traumatic incident reduction, 101–102
  charged flow, 100
  crossflow, 98, 101–103
  crossflow, 100
  inflow, 98–103
  outflow, 98, 100, 102, 103
  reflexive flow, 98, 100–103

in thematic traumatic incident reduction, 103
  during unblocking, 109. *see also* unblocking
French, Gerald, 117, 121
Freud, Sigmund, 11, 120

G

genetic counseling, 120
Gerbode, F. A., 7–8, 107, 117
group counseling, 120

I

idiosyncratic model of self, 2
  integrating trauma with, 6
Impact of Events Scale, 164
implosion, 14
indicators, 17, 131. *see also* end point
  improvement, 19
  positive, 18, 19, 21
individual counseling, 120
inflow. *see* flows
intake interview, 69
integration of traumatic event, 6
Intrusion and Avoidance scales, 164
invalidation, 107
irrational beliefs, 16

K

kinesthetic sense, 3

L

lacuna, 95
lithium, 126

M

marriage therapy, 120, 121
memory management, 6, 67, 68
metapsychology, 11, 69, 106
  substrata, 26